OXFORD MEDICAL PUBLICATIONS

Professional Development in General Practice

Professional Development in General Practice

Oxford General Practice Series • 37

Edited by

DAVID PENDLETON

and

JOHN HASLER

OXFORD NEW YORK TOKYO

OXFORD UNIVERSITY PRESS

1997

Oxford University Press, Walton Street Oxford OX2 6DP

Oxford New York
Athens Auckland Bangkok Bombay
Calcutta Cape Town Dar es Salaam Delhi
Florence Hong Kong Istanbul Karachi
Kuala Lumpur Madras Madrid Melbourne
Mexico City Nairobi Paris Singapore
Taipei Tokyo Toronto
and associated companies in
Berlin Ibadan

Oxford is a trade mark of Oxford University Press

Published in the United States
by Oxford University Press Inc., New York

© David Pendleton and John Hasler, 1997

A catalogue record for this book is available from the British Library

Library of Congress Cataloging in Publication Data
(Data available)

ISBN 0 19 262532 2

Typeset by Hewer Text Composition Services, Edinburgh

Printed in Great Britain by
Bookcraft (Bath) Ltd
Midsomer Norton, Avon

Foreword

David Metcalfe, Emeritus Professor of General Practice, University of Machester

Most doctors in practice today are the victims of their undergraduate courses! Since these were not primarily directed at learning to think clearly, they were not, properly speaking, an Education; and since they had lost the balance between acquiring knowledge, attaining skills, and developing attitudes neither were they Training. In most cases these courses were organized a round teaching and being taught, rather than on learning how to learn and then learning. These shortcomings have been compounded by over-reliance on the Multiple Choice Question format for examination, which, while being fair in the sense of test–retest and inter–observer reliability, can only test the retention of factual knowledge. Students, being intelligent people, shape their learning towards passing the next exam, so a test which, while being reliable, is not valid (in that it cannot test the acquisition of the required skills or attitudes) seriously distorts learning. Indeed the whole pattern of medical education is at odds with the pattern of clinical practice for which it is supposed to be a foundation.

- Schools admit on the basis of A-levels in scientific subjects, thereby selecting for 'convergent' or linear thinkers: clinical practice requires 'divergent' or lateral thinking.
- To get into a medical school and through it requires repeated success and a minimum of failure: clinical practice demands the ability to cope with failure.
- The basic sciences and teaching hospital medicine deal in high levels of certainty: ordinary clinical practice requires the ability to manage uncertainty.
- The course makes use of laboratories, specimens, cadavers, and non-autonomous in-patients: most clinical practice, whether specialist or GP, deals with autonomous people in their own environment.
- Students learn *on* such 'materials': clinicians work *with* sick people.
- Clinical teachers often use their vested power in teaching by the inculcation of anxiety: clinicians try to minimize the power differential with their patients and avoid generating anxiety in them.

These shortcomings in medical education not only fail to prepare the graduate adequately for practice, but also leaves him or her with some attitudinal biases which interfere with further professional and personal development. These include a preference for passive learning, in which because not active, one is not vulnerable; for learning yet more facts rather than practising skills; an assumption that one learns best from clinical specialists rather than GP colleagues, let alone teachers from disciplines such as psychology, sociology, anthropology, or economics. All of these biases are clearly visible when the patterns of postgraduate education and continuing medical education are examined, whether with regard to provision or uptake. These might be termed 'intrinsic handicaps' to development.

There is also what might be called an 'extrinsic handicap': the 'real world' does not conform to the model which furnished the basis of educational provision. Teaching hospital patients are highly selected and significantly ill. They need a precise diagnosis, which, once made, allows the rapid choice of the current 'best buy', and usually high tech treatment. The teaching specialist has been able to attain immense depth of expertise by sacrificing breadth of knowledge. The transaction of care is essentially diagnostic problem-solving in regard to a virtually passive patient. Because the choice of treatment is narrowly prescribed by the diagnosis, errors in diagnosis are regarded with much more concern than errors in treatment. For such carefully selected and seriously ill patients cost containment has, until recently, been an irrelevance. In the world of general practice people present themselves for care with minor deviations from normal health. Any of these could be, but few are, the harbingers of serious illness, yet all of which need a therapeutic response. But for specific minor illnesses and much more so for undifferentiated illness that response is not a simple response to a diagnosis. It has to take into account many features of the patient as a person, not least of which are his or her interpretations of the illness, expectations of treatment, and preferences for management. In this world errors in treatment are of greater concern than errors in 'diagnosis'. One way of summing up the difference is that in consultant practice the primary objective is precision, while in general practice the primary objective is safety.

There is one other difficulty facing the GP when he or she tries to plan continuing medical education, and that is the range of subject areas and the topics within them that have to be learned about. Because of the fact-based and disease-centred bias of conventional CME, learning is focused on specific illnesses and their treatment. But the diseases that are unfamiliar (and therefore need to be learned about) are also uncommon, and the gap between the lecture and the next patient presenting with the problem is likely to be long enough to ensure that what was taught has been forgotten. What is usually taught is the diversity of detail, while what needs to be learned is the commonality of intellectual and interpersonal skills. While a 'romantic' view of practice is that one should be left alone to do what one is best at (that is to have 'good quality' consultations) the real world does not allow this as an option: one has responsibilities to the system which enables and supports every such doctor–patient interaction.

What then needs to be learned? The answer is 'All that is needed to provide high quality care'. But what is this often used word 'quality'? In the doctor–patient interaction, whether episodic/acute or long term/chronic it has four components. Firstly it must be **safe** (risks must be minimized) or none of the others will be achievable. Secondly it must be **humane** (it must be considerate of the ill person's feelings), or neither of the others will be achievable: dissatisfaction will lead to non-compliance or 'doctor shopping'. Thirdly it must be as **effective** as possible. Lastly it must be **economic**. Interestingly when the focus shifts to the **system** (in the GP case that is the practice) the same components apply: staff must be kept safe, they must enjoy working relationships which are enhancing (humane), they must be given every chance of doing good for the patients who give them a mandate for care (effective), and the whole thing has to be run economically (not least to allow investment in new initiatives). What has to be learned, and go on being learned, therefore, is an intellectually clear way of tackling problems, whether presented by patients or pertaining to the practice. This must pay proper attention to safety, humaneness, effectiveness, and economy. That leaves the acquisition of detailed knowledge of specific diseases to knowing where, and how to access the needed information in real time, and so allows the educational programme to address the underlying competences needed in practice.

Where 'professionals' must be 'academic' is in the development and maintainance of scepticism, a necessary defence against both 'clinical fashion' and the blandishments of the pharmaceutical industry and also the various single issue pressure groups who seek to influence the pattern of practice. This is why continuing education properly directed to the craft of medicine must respect the scientific basis of that craft.

This book takes up that challenge, using the extensive practice experience of its authors to establish and explain, often with excellent case studies, the fundamental principles on which both postgraduate training and continuing medical education should be based. These include learning together, learning with specialists rather than just from them, learning from people outside medicine, and being open to stimulation from outside the practice. Importantly we should learn to see and organize CME as one component of an integrated programme of development which also includes audit and teamwork, rather than something the doctors 'go off on their own for'.

To our wives, Jennifer and Lindsay,
with thanks and with love.

Preface

By the mid-1990s there were an increasing number of stories of low morale and stress amongst British general practitioners. Ironically, this was at a time when changes in medical care were gradually propelling primary care to a central role in health care. Indeed the general practitioners of the 1950s (many of whom were also demoralized but for different reasons) would have been astounded if they had been able to foresee how pivotal general practice would become.

Some of the problem was related to a Government contract imposed insensitively. Indeed the style and speed of the changes were more of a problem than some of the content. But some of the problem was about a profession struggling to come to terms with the need for more accountability. The way in which doctors worked with each other and with other disciplines became more important as did the support mechanisms outside the practice.

Traditional continuing medical education with its emphasis on content determined by providers and where the participants were often passive became less and less relevant. In its place other activities have sprung up where the learner and her or his agenda become more important and where the emphasis is on behaviour change and personal development rather than the mere acquisition of knowledge.

The two editors have been intimately involved in many of these changes. One of us has been immersed in his own practice and on the national scene in education and teamwork for three decades. The other has been a keen observer of general practice and involved in much of its new thinking. Between us we have first-hand knowledge of much that is described in these pages.

This book has been written primarily for British general practice but there is much here that is relevant to primary care in other countries. It has been written in the hope that it can contribute to the continuing emergence of general practice as a discipline and in recognition that general practice is indeed the key to a successful health care system.

Oxford
Bristol
March 1996

J.H.
D.P.

Contents

xii *Contents*

Part III

Contributors

Richard Flew. General Practitioner, Maidenhead; Associate Adviser in General Practice, Oxford.

John Hasler. General Practitioner, Sonning Common; Regional Postgraduate Adviser and Honorary Senior Clinical Lecturer in General Practice, University of Oxford.

Peter Havelock. General Practitioner, Bourne End; Associate Adviser in General Practice, Oxford.

Jacky Hayden. General Practitioner, Bury; Regional Postgraduate Adviser in General Practice, Manchester.

Tim Huins. General Practitioner, Berinsfield; Associate Adviser in General Practice, Oxford.

Jennifer King. Psychologist, Director OPUS Consulting Ltd (Management Consultants UK and Hong Kong).

Martin Lawrence. General Practitioner, Chipping Norton; University Lecturer in General Practice, University of Oxford.

Lesley Millard. Medical Teaching Development Adviser, Faculty of Medicine, University of Southampton; Assistant Adviser (Education), South Thames (East) Regional Advisory Team in General Practice.

David Pendleton. Psychologist, Director Opus Consulting Ltd (Management Consultants UK and Hong Kong).

Roger Pietroni. General Practitioner, London; Associate Adviser in General Practice, North Thames (West).

Theo Schofield. General Practitioner, Shipston-on-Stour; RHA Lecturer in General Practice, University of Oxford.

David Whillier. General Practitioner, Paddock Wood.

Andrew Willis. General Practitioner, Northampton.

Part I

1 The need for professional development

John Hasler

General practice is changing out of all recognition. The pace of development is now breathtaking and primary medical care is beginning to move into a key position in the NHS in Britain in a way that few GPs would have dreamed of forty years ago. Yet, as the scope and possibilities increase, many doctors report disillusionment and stories of low morale abound. Somehow it seems that the needs of doctors are not being met. This chapter examines those needs and how they have arisen and argues that the present form of CME is largely inappropriate and outdated.

THE DEVELOPMENT OF GENERAL PRACTICE

The birth of the National Health Service saw general practitioners largely ousted from the hospital service which seemed to be gaining momentum. As a result many doctors (both specialists and generalists) believed that primary medical care had had its day and the picture for general practice was bleak.

But gradually things began to assume a rosier hue. The College of General Practitioners was formed and with it a journal devoted exclusively to general practice. District nurses and health visitors became attached to practices thereby stimulating the growth of primary care teams (Swift and McDougall 1964) The 1966 contract enabled significant numbers of practice nurses and administrative staff to be employed: the erection of satisfactory premises now became a realistic option. General Practitioners became more confident and began to take over the supervision of much chronic disease, whilst developments in prevention became widespread (Fowler *et al.* 1988). Computers began to appear and by the end of the eighties general practice was a popular career choice for young doctors. Apart from the increasing scope of general practice, it had remained relatively undisturbed for 25 years: in comparison, the hospital service and the health authorities had gone through a number of upheavals and undoubtedly this was another factor in attracting medical graduates to general practice.

The early nineties

Seen from the Government's viewpoint, the considerable advances made by some practices and reasonable progress made by many others were outweighed by the complacency of some and the inadequacy of a few. Against a rising tide of consumerism and spurred on by a Thatcherite policy of encouraging competition and breaking the monopolies of professions, the Government (after a relatively short private review of the NHS) introduced a number of revolutionary changes. The most significant from the viewpoint of general practice were the 1990 contract, and the purchaser–provider split whereby health authorities and fundholding practices placed contracts for hospital care, rather than the former providing this care. The main effect of the contract was to strengthen the obligations of the general practitioner and to require him or her to carry out certain activities. Included in it was a postgraduate education allowance which was paid in return for attendance at approved courses.

   Also included from 1990 was a requirement for medical audit to be undertaken by all doctors, whether in hospital or general practice. For the latter, Medical Audit Advisory Groups (MAAG) were set up, largely composed of GPs but technically answerable to the General Manager of the Family Health Services Authority (FHSA). These MAAGs were faced with a challenge. On the one hand they needed to ensure that all practices were undertaking some form of audit. On the other hand the profession considered it important that details of activities remained confidential and a potential tension existed between managers and MAAG chairmen.

THE NEEDS TODAY

A number of features of practice which create potential difficulties for doctors can now be identified.

The knowledge explosion

Medical knowledge is advancing rapidly and no doctors can carry all relevant information in their heads. This applies particularly to prescribing and drug interactions but also to new investigations, differential diagnoses and the like. Related to this are the development of protocols and management plans for various problems. Medical journals and newspapers flood through the letter box along with guidance sheets from all manner of organizations and urgent communications from the UK Government's Chief Medical Officer. Anyone who attempts to read a small proportion finds the effort soon has to be abandoned. Moreover there is no logical means of choosing what to read and which papers are a priority. Most communications end up crammed into drawers and filing cabinets or thrown into the waste paper basket. Is it any wonder that doctors feel both anxious and guilty? They are drowning in paper.

New approaches to care

In parallel with the increase in relevant knowledge, doctors are handing over some of their work to others. Most organized preventive care is now done by nurses as is a large amount of follow-up care for long term diseases such as asthma, diabetes, and hypertension (Hasler 1994). Practice managers have taken over the majority of administrative tasks in many practices. Deputizing services and co-operatives provide a significant amount of out of hours work. Much primary health care is given by other people.

New roles for the doctor

Whilst some clinical work is done by others, general practitioners now find themselves in the role of business manager, negotiator, and planner. The introduction of fund holding practices has thrown doctors into responsibilities for managing large budgets and negotiating with hospital managers. Whilst many family doctors have taken to this with relish, others are disconcerted and worried that business activities and medicine are not easy bedfellows. On top of that, advertising is now permissable and practices are starting to face competition from other practices and other forms of primary care.

New skills for the doctor

Apart from the new roles for doctors, there are specific new skills required. New technology and information systems are widespread and all doctors in the future will need keyboard skills and know how to access information through CD-ROM and computer links. On the management side all doctors have to understand what makes teams successful and how to relate and negotiate with colleagues.

The world around

As if all this were not enough, the context in which general practice functions is changing too. The introduction of the citizens' and patients' charters has highlighted the need for practices to be sensitive and respond to patients' needs and demands. Competition and market forces are encouraged and general practitioners are feeling external pressures from Government, health authorities, and patients. It is not surprising that stress levels are reported to be rising.

Given all these changes and demands, what is on offer to help general practitioners cope and flourish?

POSTGRADUATE AND CONTINUING
MEDICAL EDUCATION

In the early sixties it was recognized that journals, medical societies, and day to day activities were not enough to ensure that general practitioners continued their education adequately. There were no major criticisms of the medical school curriculum and so it was assumed that what family doctors needed primarily was the means to keep up to date. Postgraduate medical centres started to appear (Lister 1968) and by the early seventies postgraduate deans were appointed in each region to oversee and co-ordinate all aspects of postgraduate and continuing education for all — both specialists and general practitioners. General practice constituted by far and away the biggest single discipline and partly because it was widely scattered and needed co-ordinating (and partly because all deans were — and virtually still are — chosen from the ranks of specialists), regional advisers in general practice were appointed on a sessional basis to the deans' staff.

Their first (and main) preoccupation for the next two decades was to establish and develop vocational training schemes throughout the country. This major exercise had two important consequences. First, it set the pioneer general practitioners thinking about what the curriculum should be and, by inference, what skills, knowledge, and attitudes were required by the general practitioner (Royal College of General Practitioners 1972). It became all too apparent how far the medical schools were not only falling short of the mark but also could be creating problems for those students destined for general practice (McCormick 1979).

Second, since general practitioners were paid to teach, regional advisers and their colleagues realized that they needed to acquire appropriate educational skills. Within a relatively few years, there were many general practitioners who had become proficient in writing educational objectives, assessing trainees' attributes, and running small groups. Approximately a quarter of all practices became teaching practices and it was largely here that the doctors realized that to be an effective general practitioner, something much more than merely updating was needed. Special skills in communication, management, and audit were required, which sometimes involved modifying attitudes acquired earlier in the doctor's career.

Meanwhile continuing medical education (CME) was continuing largely as it had done for many years. Consultants gave lunch time or evening lectures to those general practitioners who attended the postgraduate centres. The new skills being acquired by trainees often went unnoticed. Whilst no-one could doubt the enthusiasm of most of the speakers and audience, there was little investigation into the cost-effectiveness of what was happening or how far doctors changed their behaviour as a result. Clinical Tutors who co-ordinated educational activities at district level (always specialists in the early years) were ambivalent for a long time about whether they should be informed amateurs or educational experts and generally did the work over and above their work as a hospital consultant. Regional Advisers in General Practice took little interest in CME by comparison with vocational training.

1990 AND ONWARDS

The 1990 contract shattered this state of affairs. General practitioners wishing to qualify for the new postgraduate educational allowance (PGEA) had to attend a minimum number of approved sessions each year. This approval had to be given by the Regional Advisers in General Practice, who had to set up systems of application and monitoring. Whereas the regional advisers had course organisers in each district to run vocational training, no such people existed for CME. At the time GP tutors did exist but their status and remuneration took a further three years to resolve.

The number of activities for which approval was sought climbed steadily and the volume and diversity of applicants created some problems for the advisers. The sessions spilled out of the postgraduate centres into hotels and practices. A significant number were run by the pharmaceutical industry raising questions about educational bias.

Practice based activities ranged from traditional fare provided by visiting experts to workshops for the staff. In postgraduate centres, GPs generally had to pay, whereas pharmaceutical company presentations in hotels came free, often with a meal attached. Because of the number, monitoring the educational value of most of these meetings was impossible. Furthermore, each meeting had to be allocated to one of three categories (Disease Management, Service Management, or Health Promotion) and because of the nature of many activities, a decision one way or the other was often difficult.

Advisers and GP Tutors became aware quite soon that, in spite of a large amount of activity, there were serious concerns about what was on offer in CME and, more importantly, how effective most of it was.

A mismatch of provision versus need

It has now dawned on a number of people that courses, which for many doctors remain largely as they have done for decades, no longer meet the needs identified above. Indeed, the word 'course' is in itself increasingly inappropriate. Most of them consist of lectures and seminars where knowledge is imparted by experts even though the recipients are already drowning in factual knowledge. And whilst attending a lecture may make the members of the audience feel good (if it is presented competently) there is little evidence that much is retained, or if retained, acted upon.

If we are to move forward a number of things need to happen. First, some means must be found of identifying the development needs of practices and the individuals who work there. This requires them to work out clear aims and objectives from which a sense of direction can be deduced. Merely asking people what they want to learn does not usually produce much in the way of an answer.

Second, once the needs are clear it is possible to focus on the most important issues so priority can be given to those matters that need it. If the members of the team are having difficulty working together, it may be more urgent to sort it out than undertaking some clinical knowledge updating.

Third, practices need to know that their efforts are bearing fruit. The members need to have built-in systems that demonstrate what progress is being made and where the next activities are needed.

These changes mean that education has to be turned on its head. The people who will determine the programme are the participants and learners — not the tutors. Furthermore the issues become much wider than traditional education — they are to do with the way in which practices and individuals survive, develop, and move on.

The future

There is now a recognition that the needs of doctors' professional development must be met in a much more imaginative and varied way. Furthermore activities need to be better planned and co-ordinated: it needs too to be much more clearly linked with audit than CME has been up to now. In Part II many of these new approaches are described. But first we need to understand something of what professional development means.

REFERENCES

Fowler, G Fullard, E and Gray, J. A. M. (1988). The extended role of practice nurses in preventive health care. In: *The nurse in family practice*. (A. Bowling and B. Stilwell, eds). Scutari, London.

Hasler, J. C. (1994). *The primary health care team*. Royal Society of Medicine Press, London.

Lister, J. (1968). Regional Postgraduate Medical Centres. *British Medical Journal*, 3, 736–8.

McCormick, J. (1979). *The doctor: father figure or plumber*. pp. 24–5. Croom Helm, London.

Royal College of General Practitioners (1972). *The future General Practitioner*. British Medical Association, London.

Swift, G. and McDougall, I. A. (1964). The family doctors and the family nurse. *British Medical Journal*, i, 697.

2 Professional development in general practice

David Pendleton

INTRODUCTION

Norman Cousins is an American writer. Some years ago he contracted cancer, and was admitted to hospital. Through all of his many experiences of the illness and its treatment, he retained a writer's powers of observation and became determined to document all aspects. His case was thought to be terminal but he believed in his ability to beat the disease — and succeeded. So powerful were his accounts of his life at this time that his case became well known, first throughout the United States, and subsequently around the world.

Such stories cause consternation in some medical circles. Physicians who daily battle against such obscene diseases know cases in which fighting the disease makes a difference and those in which all attempts are futile. Some advocate an optimistic and determined war against the illness. Others seek to protect their patients from the guilt and self-blame of a hopeless battle fought and lost. Yet as potentially engrossing as this story is, it is a small detail in the account which I want to emphasize as the starting point for this chapter.

Reporting a conversation with Norman Cousins in the *British Medical Journal*, Thomasina Kushner noted Cousins' distinction between hard and soft sciences. He claimed that, as he got to know his physicians over several years, they had told him of their own views about health care and their preparation for it. In medical school, they had been told that hard sciences were subjects such as physiology, pharmacology, and biochemistry. Soft subjects were psychology, sociology, and ethics.

Some years into their professional practice, however, the same physicians reflected ironically on the fact that conventional wisdom in the hard subjects had changed significantly, whereas the insights gained from the so-called soft subjects had persisted. So which, they asked, were really the hard subjects and which the soft?

This chapter will explore the similarities and differences between medical training and medical practice and will pose the question of the relevance of medical school models, which are essentially academic, to the experience of professional life in practice. It will go on to question the needs of the practising doctor for professional development and the ways in which Continuing Medical Education seeks to respond to these needs. It will conclude with the description of possible alternatives which might better suit the professionals' needs.

THE ACADEMIC AND THE PROFESSION

Those who have worked in both the academic world and in that of professional practice will be struck by their differences and by the extent to which those differences are both intriguing and disturbing. They certainly make the transition from one world to the other far from straightforward. The differences are less marked in the medical context where, it might be argued, doctors are trained rather than educated, but the point is still relevant.

Doctors are trained and qualify just once. From that point on in their careers, they can take life and death decisions with no attempt being made to reassess their continuing competence. As medical knowledge moves on, the matter of keeping their professional knowledge and skills up to date is left to the voluntary arrangements of Continuing Medical Education (CME). Inducements are made in the form of payment for attending a minimum of sessions, but this is not compulsory.

Given the seriousness of their role and the potential for calamity, we might expect their eager attendance at CME. Yet this is not the case. Most doctors do the minimum. If we make the fair assumption that most doctors are well motivated, there must be a mismatch between their needs and the education that is provided. These differences may concern the subject matter or the methods employed.

CME frequently uses the approaches and techniques of medical school training. It favours knowledge acquisition and the most efficient methods for this include listening to lectures and reading journals. General practice continuing education has developed some new and different approaches but the hard-pressed general practitioner has to make critical choices. The most basic choice is between seeing more patients or attending CME in the hope that subsequent consultations might be more effective. Then there is the matter of CME topic — paediatrics or geriatrics, asthma or AIDS, minor surgery or family therapy?

In order for the professional to take time out from the practice, the benefits of the investment of time need to be considerable — and to out-weigh the costs. And in this calculation, all factors are weighed — topic, methods, duration, payment, convenience, risk, and the like. If, on balance, there is a positive cost-benefit, most people will opt to take part.

The practitioner is particularly keen to evaluate the matter of relevance and applicability. And it is here that he or she encounters some significant differences between his or her needs and the topics and approaches used. Adrian Furnham and I have been fascinated by these differences for some time and have written about them often (e.g. Furnham and Pendleton 1991). The general case is outlined in Table 2.1.

Table 2.1 Some differences between academic and professional approaches

	Academic	Professional
Major aim	Insight and knowledge	Action to solve a problem
Urgency	Low	High
Cost-benefit analysis	Irrelevant	Crucial
Principal quality criterion	Elegance	Practicality
Usual source of insight	Own research, others' experience	Others' research, own experience
Level of complexity	High	Low
Means of persuasion	Theory backed by data	Data backed by argument
Preferred medium of presentation	Written	Face to face
Personality type most valued	Introvert	Extrovert
Method for dealing with uncertainty	Statistical	Personal

The most important difference between the two worlds is that their aims are different. The academic is seeking insight — to understand the nature and causes of things, irrespective of the use to which that insight may be put. It is sufficient in and of itself. The professional is only interested in that subset of understanding which is relevant to the problem which he or she is currently seeking to solve or manage.

Even in these increasingly cost-conscious days, academics are rarely concerned about the *time* their endeavours may take since other considerations take priority. It would be far better for an academic to rewrite a book completely, for example, and go beyond a publisher's deadline than to have the book flawed by a (perceived) lack of quality. The professional is expected to balance both quality and time and deliver both to an agreed quality standard and an agreed budget of time and money. Faced with the same dilemma as the academic, the professional would be expected, firstly, to give priority to the client's perception of quality, secondly to negotiate how the overrun of time and money was to be managed, and thirdly to resist the temptation to raise the quality of the end result beyond that required by the circumstances.

Cost-benefit analysis is also dealt with differently. When the aim is insight or understanding, greater understanding is better by definition and any incremental improvement is worth having. To distinguish between any two matters is appropriate, however small the distinction may be. Cost involved and time taken are relatively unimportant. The professional world requires that the cost of activity is born either directly by the client or absorbed by the professional. The latter represents an opportunity cost. Thus the relationship between cost and benefit has to be faced at all times and may lead to very different actions being taken.

The **principal quality criterion** in each world differs. The academic world has many well defined quality criteria which are a part of its history and philosophy. Academic quality criteria include logical consistency, precision, and verifiability. The quality criterion which tends to be uniquely emphasized, however, is the principal of parsimony which is well understood and favours contributions which are elegant. Professionals are generally employed to help find solutions or to help manage a situation more effectively. Above all, their contributions must work. After that, there are considerations of cost, time, and the quality of communication between the professional and the client. But the principal consideration is practicality.

The academic gains *insight* from his or her research, whether this is literature research or empirical research. The researcher is typically a third person, dispassionate and uninvolved. The personal experience which informs academic endeavour is usually that of other people. In the professional world, the reverse is true. Generally, the professional is drawing on a great deal of personal experience and has to guard against becoming almost totally anecdotal by checking his or her experience against the available research literature.

Falsifiability is a key academic principle which inevitably produces *complexity*. Once an idea, theory, or hypothesis has been proposed, the required task of all academic contributors is to show that all or part of it is false. This tends to complicate that which was originally simple. Kuhn's (1962) ideas about the progress of science suggest that there will indeed be simplicity again as the original idea or theory becomes so complex that it is unsustainable and it is discarded in favour of a new theory or idea. But the state of complication lasts a good deal longer than that of re-simplification with the consequence that, at any given point of academic endeavour, the current state of a theory or idea will be complex. The professional world has a low tolerance for complexity, not simply for that which is untrue.

Persuasiveness is a property of the theory and the data for the academic. The ideas persuade, not the individual. This has not always been so. Those who have wandered through the Oxford Examination Schools will have noticed the school of Astronomy and Rhetoric implying that the force of the argument may have been all that the early astronomers had at their disposal when astronomical measurement was crude. The professional is frequently to be found in the same position as the early astronomers. Physicians are well aware of the difficulties of generalizing population data to individual patients. They typically have to offer careful research done elsewhere and a keen argument to support their recommendations.

It is not surprising, therefore, that the professional's *preferred medium of presentation* is face-to-face, where the full power of the argument can be experienced. The academic publishes, hoping that those whom he or she wishes to influence will read the journals. If the academic audience has a dispute with the originator of a paper, they will write to the journal or publish a contradictory paper. The professional, having to compete with other pressing demands on the client's time, has to deal with objections as they arise so that a solution may be implemented quickly.

Not surprisingly, the academic's preferred *personality type* is introverted, and better suited to scholarship. The professional world favours extroverts, possibly better suited to dealing with people.

The most painful difference, however, is the *method of dealing with uncertainty*. The academic deals with uncertainty by addressing it explicitly and setting limits to it. The doubt which surrounds the applicability of an academic research study to the general population can be estimated and the confidence intervals can be calculated. That having been done, the matter is dealt with.

The professional is frequently in a different position. The quantity and quality of the available information brought to bear on a problem is weighed carefully but there is rarely a simple deduction which will solve the problem or manage it more effectively. The professional's judgement is sought by the client and any doubt, whether or not it is discussed, is largely dealt with by the professional personally. It is the principal source of stress in professional life.

Doctors have come to resolve this in part by sharing their uncertainty with the patient. They will honestly admit when they do not know what to do and will invite the patient to express a view, or will invite them to do nothing since nothing has been incontrovertibly demonstrated to work. This is still dealing with the uncertainty personally — albeit now interpersonally. It is certainly not the same as the academic possibility of discharging the matter of uncertainty by citing a specified confidence interval in the absence of a pressing case.

THE PROBLEMS OF
CONTINUING MEDICAL EDUCATION

Continuing Medical Education is poorly attended and the medical journals are merely skimmed, at best, by most doctors. These facts have lead the Government to introduce a new contract for medical practitioners in the National Health Service which requires them to attend CME in order to earn a small proportion of their salary.

Principally concerned with professional matters, most doctors want to improve the quality of their actions (their practice) as directly as possible. They are concerned to maximize the return on their investments — in this case, their investment of time. They will inevitably be more interested in investing an hour in CME, the faster and the broader its likely impact on their practice. This is a matter of cost-benefit analysis based on the likely yield of the activity.

A typical cost-benefit (yield) analysis in continuing medical education is provided in Table 2.2 (Pendleton 1990)

Table 2.2 Cost-benefit (yield) analysis for Continuing Medical Education

	Time cost high	Time cost low
Narrow benefit	Reading most articles in medical journals or attending most postgraduate lectures	Reading review articles or attending update lectures
Broad benefit	Attending Balint training	Video-based skills training

Maximum yield is defined here as having a low cost in terms of time and broad benefit or impact on practice. Video-based skills training makes a difference on every subsequent consultation, and requires just three days — a sound investment and has been extremely well received. Large numbers have taken part, it is now a feature of most Vocational Training Schemes in General Practice and books on this topic sell well.

Balint Training is a form of psychotherapeutically based reflection on practice in peer groups with a leader. It has a broad effect on practice but the training typically lasts for years. It has a following and a society exists for its adherents. Its yield, being broad but slow, would be classified as medium. Similarly, medium yield would describe attendance at update lectures or reading review articles in journals. But, since the absolute time involved in this activity is low compared with Balint Training and since the risk is low, more people take part in it.

The lowest yield of all is that which is associated with the most common media for Continuing Medical Education — journal articles and postgraduate lectures which are usually so narrow in their focus that it takes a great deal of time and effort to cover significant areas of a doctor's work. Thus, not surprisingly, CME is poorly attended and most journals are poorly read. This is not a failure of motivation on the part of the doctors, it is a failure of insight on the part of the providers of CME. They have based their activity on the traditional academic aims, media, and methods, when their audience is professional. They have also omitted the cost-benefit analysis of their work as perceived by their potential audience.

PROFESSIONAL DEVELOPMENT

Attempts to enhance the professional standards of practitioners are to be welcomed by all concerned with medical care — including the practitioners themselves — but they will be carefully selected on the basis of need. Busy professionals will tend to be highly selective, wishing to take the easiest steps to the enhancement of their standards of care. And there are many ways in which professional development can take place using methods which are appropriate to practice. Many are outlined in subsequent chapters of this book.

All of the techniques which are potentially most helpful will be broad in their impact on practice and will take relatively short periods of time to have their effect. Such matters will cover techniques for developing either individuals or entire practices.

Individual development might be achieved using such approaches as:

- Peer review
- Focused audit
- Action learning
- Video-based feedback on the consultation
- Joint working

Practices might be developed by:

- Strategic planning
- Team building

Techniques for individual development

Peer review

Initiatives such as the Royal College of General Practitioners' 'What sort of doctor?' are both ambitious and in the best traditions of professional development. This is one of the most powerful peer review methods. It requires practising general practitioners to visit and assess the work of a peer, in the setting of his or her own practice, against professionally established and published criteria.

The outcome is a report and a challenging conversation with the doctor to identify those features of his or her work which seemed to be of a high standard, and those where improvement could be made.

Doctors who have undertaken such reviews have found that not only receiving but also carrying out such reviews are each beneficial activities in their own right. This is a method which has still to be widely adopted but the Oxford Region's Vocational Training scheme in General Practice has a similar method in place for reviewing its training practices. (For more on this, see Chapter 7.) It is also the basis of the Fellowship by Assessment of the UK Royal College of General Practitioners.

Focused audit

In contrast with Practice Activity Analysis (PAA) which analyses actions in the absence of any *a priori* standard, Focused Audit would establish a standard first and then seek to understand what caused the standard to be implemented or undermined in the practice of an individual doctor.

For example, there may be five preconditions which should be met for a prescription of a particular medication. Focused audit would simply pull out the consultation notes of the last 10 or 20 scripts for the specified medication and investigate how often these conditions were met. The learning takes place in understanding the reasons why action is taken which is acknowledged to be inappropriate and discussing ways of bringing the standard and the behaviour into alignment.

Action learning

Action learning (Revans 1982) is a means of developing expertise in fields which are new to all taking part. Typically, a group of professionals will decide to tackle a new area of work and will agree how to structure their activities and reflect on their experience in a way which ensures that as much is learned as fast as possible by all members of the group. Occasionally, action learning groups find it easier to make progress when they have an external facilitator.

Video-based feedback on consultations

This technique brings fast results when it is based on real consultations and evaluation takes place against clear and mutually agreed criteria. It is becoming widely used in vocational training and is one of the most potentially helpful means of continuing professional development. See Pendleton *et al.* (1984) and Chapter 4 in this volume.

Joint working

The opportunity to learn from others is a feature of partnership and yet it is infrequently used. Similar opportunities present themselves to learn from specialists. Ben Pomryn was an unusual psychiatrist who conducted pioneering work of this kind in the 1970s and 80s, regularly visiting general practitioners to conduct joint surgeries with them. In this way he would develop their expertise in dealing with the psychological aspects of practice — whether dealing with patients' needs or doctors'. By the time of his death he had provided a model for others to use. See Chapter 5 in this volume.

Techniques for practice development

Strategic planning workshops

These are opportunities for practices to raise their eyes from the present day and focus on the future. The key questions to be asked here are twofold: what kind of practice do we want to become and how are we going to achieve it? These workshops are best facilitated so that awkward matters (and individuals?) can be confronted safely. They may be confined to the partners or may involve everyone if that is the way the practice runs. Pendleton (1990) first proposed these workshops and Chapter 3 in this volume describes how they work. The workshops reveal the values which underpin most of the decisions taken in the practice. They may also demonstrate that the partnership does not satisfy the preconditions for association — namely a shared vision of the future to which all are committed.

Team building

Teams, like gardens, do not generally do well without attention to their needs and their growth. Team building is a deliberate and systematic attempt to provide for the team's needs. Teams tend to pass through a number of growth stages (known as Forming, Storming, Norming) before achieving maturity (Performing). These various stages are well documented, but rather less is known about the evolution of established teams.

Nonetheless, it appears that occasional attention to such matters as planning can become ideal settings for team building. The involvement of team members in making decisions which affect them tends to increase their commitment to the decisions made. This is a general principle of decision making (Janis and Mann 1977). Strategic Planning Workshops have team building as a by-product. Other shared activities will serve a similar purpose — even if they are social — but involvement in structured activities with opportunities for structured feedback and reflection seem to work best.

ESTABLISHING THE AGENDA FOR PROFESSIONAL DEVELOPMENT

In order to develop practitioners and practices to best advantage, more is required than the introduction of techniques such as those outlined above. There needs to be a significant re-focusing of CME, and the creation of an appropriate infrastructure comprising established posts, systems, funding, and approaches. This is a theme to which we will return in Part III of this book in which we consider the features of a Blueprint for professional development in the twenty-first century. It is appropriate here, however, to consider the matter of how professional development agendas may be set — both for individuals and practices.

In this context, the key is to remember that professional development's principal aim is to improve practice — and it is in the world of practice that the agenda is best set through a series of diagnoses. The entire cycle of activity is shown overleaf in Fig. 2.1

One of the difficulties facing medical practitioners currently is the absence of guidance on development needs. The problem is not that individuals cannot choose well, but rather that the basis of choice is unclear. If we accept that the individual practitioner is seeking to be effective in a specific context of a practice, then the overall practice strategic plan would be an ideal starting point. The problem is that most practices do not have such a thing. What is more, there are relatively few places they could turn to find help in the creation of such a plan (for more on this, see Chapter 3 in Part II and all of Part III at the end of this book).

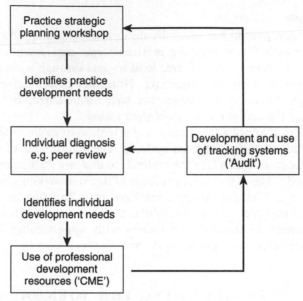

Fig 2.1   The professional development cycle

The strategic plan would comprise a number of elements including the current strengths and limitations of the practice, and the areas in which they need to make progress in order to realize their aims. In other words, the practice's development needs would have been identified along with individual accountabilities for making progress in these areas — and this already creates an agenda for professional development in a few specified areas.

Additional use of diagnostic methods for individual practitioners further develops the agenda. The use of peer review methods, or consultation analysis, or even paper and pencil tests in relevant areas helps individuals and groups to pinpoint the professional development activities which are most relevant to their needs. Thus, instead of avoiding CME or partaking in it on the basis of weakly held preferences, busy practitioners would be able to specify the precise help they need.

The advantages of this for the individual practitioners are easy to see, but there are additional advantages for those currently charged with responsibility for providing CME — the GP Tutors — and those who are involved as Audit Facilitators. GP Tutors are frequently faced with considerable doubt as to what activities to offer. Audit Facilitators have to persuade and cajole often-reluctant practitioners to audit their work without a clear rationale. The development and use of tracking systems allows the techniques of audit to be applied in their proper context — the achievement of aims, progress towards which needs to be monitored.

In the model proposed here, the development of practices and individuals may be addressed and the activities of GP Tutors and Audit Facilitators may be brought together and given their rightful place. If CME and Audit are ever to be more than mere adjuncts to practice, they need to be integrated into the context of a continuing cycle of professional development.

REFERENCES

Furnham, A. and Pendleton, D. (1991). The academic consultant. *Journal of General Management*, **17** (2), 13–19.

Janis, I. and Mann, I. (1977). *Decision making: a psychological analysis of conflict, choice and commitment*. Free Press, New York.

Kuhn, T. (1962). *The structure of scientific revolutions*. University of Chicago Press.

Pendleton, D. (1990). *The educational process: methods and opportunities*. Paper presented at BMS Conference on Continuing Medical Education in General Practice, Dublin, February 1990.

Pendleton, D., Schofield, T., Tate, P., and Havelock, P. (1984). *The consultation: an approach to learning and teaching*. Oxford University Press.

Revans, R. (1982). *The origins and growth of action learning*. Chartwell Bratt, London.

Fig. 2.1 The professional development cycle.

Part II

3 Shaping the future with Strategic Planning Workshops

Jennifer King and Richard Flew

> 'Shaping strategic success requires organisations to recognise and articulate those values that drive its decisions and to disseminate those values throughout the organisation'
> (Pfeiffer 1989)

INTRODUCTION

The demands of the new general practice contract have provoked changes in roles, expectations, and responsibilities in general practice — changes which have exposed both strengths and weaknesses in many practice teams. Practices which were able to function under the 'old order' have found that the changes highlighted differences in values which in some cases posed real difficulties for the functioning of the practice. For other practices, the changes have presented a positive opportunity to move forward — to adopt a more business-like approach and to deal with changes by anticipating them rather than reacting to events. In either event, practices have needed increasingly to re-examine their existing values and roles and to define clearer goals for the future.

Chapter 2 highlights two themes in professional development in general practice — development of individuals and development of practices. The focus of this chapter is on practice development. Instead of being reactive to change, practices can choose to shape their professional development by formulating and implementing a strategic plan.

Practices may find the very idea of a strategic plan to be alien and daunting, but of course it is neither. Strategic planning means simply creating a programme of actions that will change the practice over a specified period of time from the way it is now, to the way its members want it to be. This chapter illustrates how strategic planning workshops can be a valuable means of developing practices. It describes a particular approach and cites a case study of a practice which, despite working well, wanted to be more able to manage change more positively — to move, in effect, from competence to excellence.

The chapter begins with a description of a strategic planning tool known as 'Force-Field Analysis'. It presents a case study to show how the tool worked in practice. The chapter goes on to summarize the most important steps and guidelines for effective strategic planning. The final section identifies the critical issues highlighted by this method — namely, leadership, vision, accountability, and change management.

CONTRIBUTION TO PRACTICE

The planning process: 'force-field analysis'

The approach known as force-field analysis seeks to arrive at a clearer idea of the future by comparing aspirations with reality and then analysing the 'forces' that are working to help or hinder these aspirations. The strategic plan seeks to remove the hindrances and capitalise on the helping factors. Force-field analysis can be represented diagramatically (see Fig. 3.1).

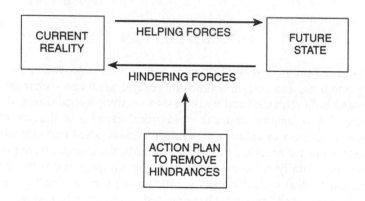

Fig. 3.1   Force-field analysis.

Stage one: identifying the vision (future state)

The first objective of the planning process is to help the practice team produce a clear statement (or series of statements) defining its goals for the future — commonly known as a Mission Statement. Its mission embodies the practice's values and is a rallying cry for all of its members. Members who do not subscribe to these broad aims will feel very uncomfortable in the practice and may even not belong in it at all.

This is a key stage in strategic planning. It is often said that an organization's success depends largely on clarity of mission. Two key questions need to be asked: (1) What kind of practice do we want to be? (2) How are we going to achieve it? This kind of understanding must be widespread and shared in order to develop commitment and loyalty to the practice and its success. The mission — or set of goals — must be clearly stated if it is to be accomplished effectively. Ambiguous statements leave room for dodging the issues and for lack of accountability. The vision of the future should at this stage be very ambitious and not held back by current problems.

Stage two: current reality

This stage is much briefer and involves taking each of the practice ideals identified in Stage one and comparing it with what currently happens. This gives a clearer sense of how close or far the practice is from its vision.

Stage three: helping and hindering forces

The practice identifies the factors that are working in its favour to help it achieve its ideals. This is useful in helping to highlight the strengths of the team. It is important to focus on aspects that are *currently true* rather than a 'wish list'. It gives a clearer picture of what the team can build upon and develop.

The hindrances are also identified (again, those that are currently true but perhaps also some potential obstacles). The list of hindrances is then further divided into those that are out of the immediate control of the practice, those that can be rectified but slowly, and those that can be quickly overcome. Those out of its control should be ignored for the purpose of formulating a strategy. The focus should be on areas where constructive actions can be taken. It is these proposed actions which form the basis of the final stage.

Stage four: action planning (the strategy)

The action plan is, in effect, a definition of both strategy and tactics. This stage focuses on the main hindrances and should identify specifically how each one should be overcome. The recommended actions should be highly specific — defining *what* should be done, how, *by whom*, *by when*, and where possible how progress will be *measured*.

CASE STUDY

Background to case study

A number of particularly significant changes prompted this particular practice to re-evaluate its future needs. It must be emphasized, however, that this was not a practice in trouble. As an old established practice of six partners, it had an opportunity to change to become more effective. For a long time its decisions had been made reactively 'riding the punches', responding quickly to external pressures. It was not one particular stimulus, but several in quick succession, that created the internal environment that stimulated this planning activity. Recent changes included:

1. A new building
2. A recent appointment of a new partner
3. Becoming fundholders
4. The new contract
5. The retirement of a long-established practice manager
6. The failure to select an appropriate practice manager

All these events, some successfully managed and some not, highlighted the lack of planning in this practice. Did everyone have a similar view of the future? Was this view communicated to others? Where was the plan for the future? Where were the skills and capabilities to make a plan? These issues are not often addressed in general practice, so experience from outside of the field of general practice was sought from two business psychologists to design and facilitate a strategic planning meeting.

Pre-contracting

The objectives of the pre-contracting stage are (1) to build rapport between the facilitator and the workshop participants, (2) to identify expectations and concerns relating to the workshop, and (3) to clarify the important issues as a basis for planning the workshop. Pre-contracting involved a series of one-to-one, confidential interviews with each participant. This is invaluable groundwork and is to be encouraged even if the facilitator is well-known to the group.

Structure of the planning meeting

An initial strategic planning meeting requires involvement from all the key decision-makers in the practice. In this case, it was agreed that the initial meeting would be restricted to partners and practice manager. In planning subsequent workshops, the practice expanded this limited number to include all members of the practice and primary health care team. The decision not to involve all members in the initial meeting was based on several reasons:
- Anxieties about the size of the practice team itself (it would involve 50 people)
- A feeling that decisions to be made at the time were more appropriate to 'Board Members' (i.e. fundholding decisions, personal partner development plans, and the introduction of a new practice manager)
- Anxieties about the process of the day (partners would be involved in a new way of looking at themselves)

Experience suggests that each practice must make the decision about who should be involved and will need to take the following issues into account.
- involving key people
- the size of the team
- the functioning of the team at that particular time
- the anxiety levels of the partners

Agreeing a vision for the future

Each individual member of the workshop group began by presenting their personal vision of the future. When these were compared it was clear that the individual visions were broadly similar. At this stage, however, considerable debate and negotiation is needed in order to arrive at a consensus vision to which all members can commit. This practice chose to express their joint vision in the following mission statement.

Patient care	We wish to anticipate and accept patients health needs and consistently provide high quality care which will promote their ability to take the best care of themselves.
A common purpose	We wish that all team members agree and work towards the same values and priorities and to understand their roles within the team.
Happiness	We wish all members of the team to be valued, appropriately trained, and work in clear roles with the respect and support of their colleagues and feel in control of their work.
Money	We wish to maximize the practice net income consistent with our other aims and distribute it equitably.
Time	We wish to ensure that the allocation of time reflects our priorities.

Arriving at a consensus vision of the future is invariably the most challenging stage of this planning process. It requires strong facilitation — preferably by someone who is not emotionally too close to the issues. It requires time and participation by all concerned. Mission statements are necessarily rather general to begin with — if they are to be implemented, they need to be qualified with highly specific statements. Vague or ambiguous wording (e.g. 'Treat the staff better'; 'spend more time with patients'; 'strengthen research activities') is open to misinterpretation. Worse, the goals may be ignored because they are not specific enough for people to act upon.

Identifying helping and hindering factors

Considerable discussion had already taken place during the previous stage of identifying the vision, when descriptions of the present state were frequently used to highlight this vision of the future. When this practice described its 'current state' in relation to the five mission statements, it was reassuring that in many areas the practice was closer to its vision that it had realized. Many helping forces were identified, including:
- Well established practice
- Loyal hard-working staff
- New facilities
- Skills of different members of the staff and partnership
- Efficient and up-to-date record system

There was also consensus about the hindering forces:
- Too many patients
- Too few appointments
- Not enough time

- Outside commitments
- Paperwork

It was interesting that a great number of these were associated with lack of information that was needed to make logical decisions. It was clear that the practice had made decisions in the past by guesswork and presumption, and in many cases, prejudice. The exercise identified these areas of ignorance so that in the next stage information could be found to enable appropriate judgements to be made.

In some cases, factors which work in favour of the team can also work against them, and vice versa — so some overlap can usually be expected in this stage. For example, many outside commitments may be a help to the practice in terms of bringing in new ideas and resources, but a hindrance in terms of time away from the practice. The findings from the psychological questionnaires (i.e. particular personality characteristics) were also included in the lists — both as helping and hindering factors.

Working relationships in the practice — a psychological analysis

The ability of any practice team to work effectively depends ultimately on the personalities of its members. Some of these personality characteristics may be acting as either helping or hindering factors to the development of the practice as a whole. This practice used psychometric (psychological measurement) methods to understand more fully the strengths within its own team as well as some of the areas which might impede smooth working relationships. Psychometric methods are becoming increasingly popular in selecting staff (King and Whitfield 1990) and their value in team-building and forming working groups is being increasingly recognized and implemented by general practitioners.

Interpreting and feeding back the results of these psychometric measures requires sensitive handling. Used appropriately, there is considerable potential benefit for teams and individuals.

Two instruments which have been used in practice team development activities for some years are the Belbin Self-Perception Inventory which analyses team roles, and the FIRO-B which explores how people interact with one another.

Belbin Self-Perception Inventory Extensive research conducted at Henley Staff College by R. Meredith Belbin (Belbin 1981) identified eight roles which made up what Belbin called a 'winning team'. These roles can be represented either by eight different people, or one person can adopt more than one role. The roles identified by Belbin are as follows:

- Chairman/Co-ordinator: co-ordinating leadership
- Plant: generator of ideas
- Monitor–Evaluator: 'sifter' of ideas
- Team worker: looks after the internal relationships

- Resource investigator: looks after the external relationships (networking)
- Implementer: loyal to the group/company/organization; will do anything required
- Completer–Finisher: ensures completion of tasks and projects

Open discussion of the results is in itself of benefit since it allows each individual to recognize and understand where he or she contributes to or detracts from the team effort. This practice, for example had a Shaper (a strong leader who acts as a driving force in a team) and a Monitor–Evaluator who sifts through ideas generated by others and decides which are worth keeping and which discarding. This can generate potential conflict with others who are less concerned with evaluating ideas and more eager to put them into practice. Thus the conflicts which had tended to arise between the Shaper and Monitor–Evaluator in this practice were explained and understood. Similarly it was recognized that in a practice which was typically involved in a variety of projects and initiatives, it was essential to have a Completer–Finisher in the team to ensure that such projects were actually completed. In this practice only one Completer–Finisher emerged and it became clear why she had felt so overloaded. It was recognized that a practice manager should be a Completer–Finisher but it would also be useful for one of the partners to adopt this role.

The information from the Belbin Self-Perception Inventory enabled the practice members to negotiate the important roles that each partner took. It also enabled issues about roles and values to be discussed in a context where all the roles have an equal value within the team.

FIRO-B (Fundamental Interpersonal Relationships Orientation — Behaviour) (Schultz 1966) Developed in the USA by Will Schutz the FIRO-B is a measure of a person's characteristic behaviour towards other people in three areas: *inclusion*, *control*, and *affection*. To illustrate these categories, Schutz presents the analogy of a group of people riding in a boat. The inclusion issue is the decision to go or not to go on the boat ride. The issue of control with the boat is who is running the engine or operating the rudder. The affection issue concerns any close relations that develop between pairs of people.

These areas are further divided into measures of *expressed* and *wanted* behaviour. For example, a common profile found in general practitioners (when answered in the context of their working relationships) is high scores on expressed inclusion (i.e outwardly sociable towards people) yet low scores on wanted inclusion (no strong need for social contact). Another characteristic profile in GPs is low scores on both expressed and wanted control — reflecting a desire neither to give nor to receive orders. This suits independent contractor status but does not predispose them to teamwork or leadership.

Partnership difficulties can often be more clearly understood by using the FIRO-B — for example, it may be the case that a partner who appears unsociable and rarely contributes to making decisions may be seen as uncommitted — whereas his FIRO-B score suggests that he is nervous of taking on responsibility and has a strong need to be liked. He fears rejection so strongly that he will not take the risk of making a mistake — either in decision-making or relationships.

The FIRO-B has one major drawback — it is fakeable. Respondents may be tempted to answer the questions in terms of how they would like to be rather than how they actually behave. For this reason it is not a useful instrument for recruitment purpose; for team development, however, there may be greater motivation to present an accurate picture of oneself. At the very least the results can stimulate valuable discussion around working relationships and in many cases can produce new insights into patterns of interaction which may be helping or hindering the team. In this particular practice the FIRO-B highlighted the following issues:

- The need for inclusion. The common profile as described above of general practitioners with high expressed inclusion (outwardly sociable) and low wanted inclusion (i.e. selective in our associations with others) was shown also within this practice. Combining that with the strong control scores begs the question 'How good was this practice at working within teams?'
- The need for control. Two partners had scores described in the FIRO-B terminology as 'Mission Impossible', i.e. not prepared to be controlled but keen to control others and to take on many responsibilities. The discussions that took place around this particular issue enabled the whole practice to understand why conflicts had arisen in the past and how best to deal with them in the future. The aim was not so much to stop all conflict, but to understand why it occurred and use it constructively.
- The need for support. The scores of at least one member of the team surprised us all in the imbalance between a low level of expressed affection and a high degree of wanted affection. The message received from partners in day-to-day activities are not always the ones that they wish us to receive. The FIRO-B has enabled support to be given in a more active way as particular needs have been highlighted.

Benefits of the psychometric measures Both these psychological instruments had their greatest value in the discussions that were stimulated by the analysis of the results. On many subsequent occasions, discussions return to the issues that arose at that time:

- Does the practice have a range of Belbin team roles, and who is fulfilling them at any one time?
- Do we always rely on one person to finish off the projects?
- Are new ideas given appropriate time and analysis?
- Is appropriate support given to individuals within the team?
- Do we recognize those under stress?

Action plan to remove hindrances

To maximize the chances of implementation, action plans should be SMART (Specific, Measurable, Achievable, Relevant, and Trackable). Following these principles, the following actions were identified:

1. To review patients' services. i.e. to analyse both the supply and the demand. The practice needed a clear understanding of the services that were actually being provided and some assessment of the needs of the practice in the future.
2. To introduce a system for personal development. This involved the introduction of an appraisal system within the practice, involving both staff and partners. It was agreed that this should be a system that enabled all members of the practice to express their views about their role within the team.
3. The development of a system of financial planning with the exploration of a profit sharing system for staff. Poor financial planning through lack of current financial information meant many decisions had been made without a clear view of how the fund was being used.
4. To explore the introduction of para-medical services into the practice. A long discussion had taken place about the role of doctors, nurses, and other paramedical services, in the practice, with a general view that much of what was being done by doctors could be better done by others.

For each of the above, one or two partners assumed responsibility and set a date for presentation of their findings and progress.

Involving the practice team

An initial planning meeting must always address the issue of how best to communicate its conclusions to the rest of the staff. A sense of ownership is crucial for a mission to be achieved. A number of strategies were discussed for how to involve other practice members:

- Repeat the exercise with a greater number of the team.
- Allow each area of the practice (nurses, receptionists, etc.) to undertake similar exercises and hope that similar statements would appear that could be amalgamated into one.
- Present the mission statement with the aim of having its value accepted by other members in the team.
- Attempt to launch a new practice by combining the mission statements and action plans with other activities to build a new environment.

Given the importance of demonstrating clear leadership and setting an example for others to follow, the final option of the launch was chosen. It was implemented in the following ways which would symbolize a new beginning:

- A new practice logo was designed and incorporated into new stationery.
- New practice leaflets were produced.

- Practice sweaters were produced for all to wear, particularly receptionists at the desk.
- Photographs of all members of the staff and partners were hung in the waiting room.

A launch date was set when the mission statement and related materials would be presented to the whole team. Reactions to the presentation were extremely positive, although regret was expressed by some over not being involved in the original planning exercise. In conclusion, and with the benefit of hindsight this was a planning exercise which helped a good practice to become better, which enabled a reactive practice to become pro-active, which helped a group of individuals to become a team, and which identified the source of leadership on the practice. It is currently a practice where individuals are respected and valued, where their needs for support and challenge are recognized, and where all share a common view of the future.

A STEP-BY-STEP GUIDE

From our experience, several questions are commonly asked about these strategic planning workshops. The following are the most frequent and some recommendations are provided for each:

Planning the workshop

Who should we use to facilitate the workshop?
Use an outside facilitator who can be more objective yet who has some understanding of general practice issues.

Do you need special qualifications to use psychometric measures?
Only qualified (Chartered) psychologists, or people trained by them or through courses run by the test publishers/distributors in the use of these measures are permitted to purchase, administer, and interpret them. Details of training for the FIRO-B are given at the end of this chapter. The use of the Belbin Inventory requires copyright permission from the author.

How long do we need to run a workshop?
Set aside at least one full day (10 to 12 hours) of uninterrupted time, preferably away from the practice. Practice 'away-days' often involve a strategic planning activity.

Who should be invited to the initial workshop?
This depends on the state of the partnership. A practice that is already working well may welcome broader involvement not only for partners but practice manager, nurse, representative, etc. Practices with major problems may prefer

to confine initial discussions to the partners. Subsequent events can involve more people once initial problems have been addressed. This is not an expression of elitism — rather it is an expression of leadership. Extremely large numbers make the event unwieldy. A group of practice members should be interviewed before the workshop to include their views.

Do we always need a pre-contracting phase?

One-to-one interviews with every workshop participant helps to allay anxieties and develop rapport with an outside facilitator. It is an important ice-breaker and saves time during the day itself. It also ensures that the critical issues are addressed.

During the workshop

How do we make sure that action plans are actually implemented?

Focus action plans on removing hindrances within the practice's control. For factors outside its immediate control, focus on ways to cope or simply accept their existence and work around them. Considerable time can otherwise be wasted on actions that are neither achievable nor realistic. Ensure that accountabilities are clear — assign actions to people and given them clear targets and ways to measure their success

How do we tell the rest of the staff about the workshop?/How much should we tell them?

Build in time towards the end to plan how to communicate the outcomes of the workshop — and especially the vision and mission — to the rest of the staff. Agree a consistent statement or policy of how you will address initial enquiries from staff about the workshop.

After the workshop

How do we keep up the momentum?

Plan a follow-up meeting to track progress against agreed targets; set a date to communicate the outcomes to the rest of the staff; consult widely on difficult issues. For example, working groups could be set up involving everyone in the practice. These groups could confer regularly and share progress.

How do we deal with cynicism from the staff?

This is usually an indication of feeling threatened and uninvolved. It might also be that previous planning initiatives have resulted in little visible benefit to the staff. Inform and consult as early and as widely as possible. Address enquiries from other practice members openly. Seek their opinions before the workshop and ensure that these views are taken into account.

CONCLUSIONS

Strategic planning is more than just a tool for developing a practice: it is an expression of leadership which establishes the principles for working — as individuals and as a team. Provided the rest of the staff are consulted and the mission and vision communicated early, the practice can move forward together (often referred to as 'alignment') committed to the same aims. The planning activity in itself can have a team-building function: it can open up channels of communication between team members and increase their awareness of the strengths and weaknesses of the team.

A critical issue which often concerns those who are proposing a strategic planning event is: who should be included? This ultimately depends upon the sort of practice you wish to be. The style of communication in Practices (as in most organisations) is likely to fall somewhere along the following continuum:

Tell............... Sell.................... Consult.................. Involve

- Partners who *tell* their staff simply announce the conclusions as a 'fait accompli' and with the expectation that they will be carried out without challenge.
- Partners who *sell* the decisions try to persuade their staff of the desirability of these decisions. Questions are actively encouraged and concern is shown for staff satisfaction. The case study above is an example of this approach.
- Partners who *consult* their staff make the final decision but only after presenting the issues to the staff and gathering their advice and opinions.
- Partners who *involve* their staff do not make the final decision — rather they define the problem, and allow majority opinion to determine the decision.

Practices will need to decide which of these methods is appropriate for their particular working climate, and be aware that the approach they choose will in itself communicate their practice values.

It is these values, inherent also in the vision and mission, which will ultimately drive the way in which the team pursues its goals. For a practice to work well these values need to be shared. The strategy which follows from these shared values will act as a basis for recruiting new staff and appraising the performance of existing staff, in the sense that all staff should be working towards the mission and in line with the practice values. Thus, the strategy becomes a means for making key decisions, managing people, and establishing a working climate.

Naturally, there are many ways of achieving a strategic plan. The practice may do it alone when they feel they have the appropriate skills, or a facilitator may be involved to help the process along. A practice may even need an outside organization to devise a strategic plan for the practice. Management consultants do this for many organizations. The approach described here is particularly well suited to general practice, however, as it is involving.

Strategic planning is a critical part of professional development in general practice. It can enable general practitioners to manage their future more pro-actively whilst retaining their responsiveness to patient and staff needs. Above all it can create a practice which can respond to change. As Scully and Byrne (1987) remarked 'The best way to predict the future is to invent it'.

NOTE

Details of training use of the FIRO-B can be obtained from:
Oxford Psychologists Press Ltd.,
Lambourne House,
311–321 Banbury Road,
Oxford, OX2 7JH,
UK.
Telephone: 01865 510203   Fax: 01865 310368

REFERENCES

Belbin, R. M. (1981). *Managerial teams. Why they succeed or fail*. Heinemann, Oxford.
King, J. and Whitfield, M. (1990). How to choose a new partner in general practice. *British Medical Journal*, **301**, 1258–60.
Pfeiffer, J. W., Goodstein, L. D. and Nolan, T. M. (1989). *Shaping strategic planning*. University Associates Inc., New York.
Schutz, W. (1966, original publication 1958). *The interpersonal underworld*. Science Behaviour Books, Palo Alto, CA.
Scully, J. and Byrne, J. A. (1987). *Odyssey: Pepsi to Apple*. Harper and Row, New York.

4 Learning consultation skills

Peter Havelock and Theo Schofield

INTRODUCTION

The consultation is central to the work of the general practitioner. It is the point at which the doctor's knowledge is applied to and shared with the patient. It can be a highly skilled communication process but unfortunately it is not always as effective as it could be. In surveys of patients' views (College of Health 1991), the consultation is always the main feature of dissatisfaction because of:
• Consultations feeling too rushed
• Problems not being understood
• Explanations being complex and too long
• Doctors not appearing to listen or pay attention

The field of doctor–patient communication has been widely researched and there is a great deal of evidence to support the factors which make or impair effective consultation. Byrne and Long (1976) in their aptly named book *Doctors talking to patients* concluded that 'the majority of GPs seem to evolve, largely by trial and error, a relatively static style of consulting'. Others researching into patient compliance have found that a static style does, not produce the required outcome for either doctor or patient.

Podell (1975) in a survey of the literature on compliance regarding hypotensive drugs concluded that one-third of patients did not follow advice, one-third followed some advice but not enough to be effective, and only one-third followed enough of their doctor's advice for it to be effective. Pendleton and Bochner (1980) found that communication difficulties for doctors occurred in a quarter of all consultations. Phillip Ley in the introduction to his book *Communicating with patients* (Ley. 1988) referring to eight articles written between 1966 and 1983 said 'Despite the attention that the techniques for improving communication have received over the last two decades or so there is no evidence that the problems of patients' dissatisfaction with communications and their often low co-operation in treatment is diminishing'.

There is no doubt that the consultation is important not only to patients but also to doctors of whom it is a major part of their working life. In all consultations there are areas that could be changed and developed to make the communication more effective for both parties. In this chapter we aim to answer two questions — that does being effective mean? What abilities are required to conduct an effective consultation? We will also examine ways in which these abilities can be developed and maintained.

HOW THE APPROACH CONTRIBUTES TO PRACTICE

There can be many reasons why patients with a problem choose to consult a doctor, rather than talk to family or friends or manage it themselves. These may include the fact that doctors are trained to diagnose 'medical' problems and prescribe treatment. One definition of effectiveness is if the diagnosis of the nature, history, and cause of the problem is correct, and the treatment appropriate. We are also well aware as general practitioners that there are many other factors that influence the decision to consult, including patients' ideas about the problem and what it might mean to them, the worries or concerns they may have, as well as the effect the problem is having on their lives. An effective consultation would therefore be one in which the doctor explores and understands all the reasons for a patient's attendance, and in which the needs of the patient are met. These needs may also include the necessity to consider at risk factors such as blood pressure or lifestyle, and continuing medical problems that the patient does not present at the time.

Various approaches

The outline above is reflected in the Patient Centred Clinical Method developed by Stewart and colleagues (Levenstein *et al.* 1986) in which they describe the doctor exploring two agendas, the medical agenda of the history of the problem and its diagnosis, and the patient's agenda of his or her experience of the illness. The strength of this model is in demonstrating the integration of these two agendas into a full understanding of the whole person and problem. This is particularly helpful for medical students who may be receiving apparently conflicting messages from clinical teachers on the one hand about 'taking' histories, and from communication skills courses on the other. Students also have to struggle to maintain their natural interpersonal skills in the face of time and other pressures in the clinical environment.

Another approach is to consider what happens after the consultation. When the patient emerges from the consulting room there are some immediate outcomes, including whether they can remember the information that they were given, whether they feel satisfied with the consultation, and whether they have any intention of following advice. The importance of these outcomes is that they influence the patient's compliance and hopefully this will lead to improvements in their health. How is this achieved in the consultation? The evidence is that while patients may report feeling more satisfied immediately after a consultation in which they are told what to do (Savage and Armstrong 1990), they are more likely to take good care of their health if they are fully informed, involved in decisions, and encouraged to take appropriate responsibility themselves. (Greenfield *et al.* 1986). Many doctors and patients take the view that being healthy does not just depend on the absence of disease but also on the ability to make informed choices and have control of one's life, including the choice of when to seek medical advice. An effective consultation can therefore be viewed as one in which patients gain the information, the involvement and the independence necessary to promote their own health.

These definitions of effectiveness and the evidence that supports them were brought together by Pendleton *et al.* (1984) as a set of Tasks to be achieved in a consultation which are set out in Table 4.1.

The wording of the last task is important as it does not attempt to dictate how individual doctors should relate to their patients or a cookbook of how they should behave. Instead it states that whatever the doctor's style, consultations in which patients can talk about their ideas and concerns, and in which information, decisions, and responsibilities are shared, are more likely to meet the patients needs and promote their health than those in which these tasks are not achieved.

Table 4.1 Seven tasks for the consultation

Task 1 To define the reasons for the patients' attendance including:
- the nature and history of the problems
- the aetiology
- the patients' ideas, concerns, and expectations
- the effects of the problems

Task 2 To consider other problems:
- continuing factors
- at risk factors

Task 3 To choose an appropriate action with the patient for each problem

Task 4 To achieve a shared understanding of the problem with the patient.

Task 5 To involve the patient in the management, and to encourage acceptance of appropriate responsibility

Task 6 To use time and resources appropriately:
- in the consultation
- in the long term

Task 7 To establish or maintain a relationship with the patient which helps to achieve the other tasks.

What does it take to be effective?

The term 'patient centred' was first used by Byrne and Long (1976) in their attempt to describe and to classify the behaviours or skills that they heard used (audiotape recordings, etc.) in general practice consultations. Behaviours that drew on the patient's knowledge and experience, such as listening, asking open questions, seeking the patient's opinion, and explaining using the patient's own words were classified as patient centred. Asking closed questions and giving instructions were examples of doctor centred behaviours. They also found that while there was a wide range of possible behaviours individual doctors had limited repertoires, and their degree of doctor or patient centredness did not vary with the nature of the problem. Faced with a patient with a suspected fracture and one with depression the doctor centred doctor would ask 'Does it hurt here?' and 'Do you wake up at 5 a.m.?', while the patient centred doctor would ask 'How does it feel?' and 'How do you sleep?'. There is no single right or wrong style and one aim in trying to become more effective is to expand the repertoire of skills and to be able to use them appropriately.

Other necessary attributes are the strategies that doctors use and the way that they make decisions in the consultation. As soon as patients start to present their problems the doctor is picking up cues and generating hypotheses which can then be tested. These hypotheses may be chosen on the basis of probability, risk, or potential treatability. The process can fail if, for example, the cues are missed, the hypotheses are inappropriate, or the information obtained inadequate to make the correct diagnosis. It is usually helpful to allow patients to tell their story in their own words without interrupting or jumping to premature conclusions. There is good evidence that if this can be done patients are more likely to tell doctors their real concerns (Buckman and Frankel 1984). Furthermore it may also help time to be used more effectively.

As well as the tasks to be achieved in consultations and the strategies and skills the doctor uses to achieve them, attributes of doctors themselves influence their effectiveness. Doctors bring their own knowledge, attitudes, beliefs, and awareness of their own feelings and reactions to their consultations. These may be influenced by a lifetime of professional or personal experience, or by events that day or in the previous consultation. They can affect consultations in a multitude of ways, for example on our willingness to explore a distressing problem or to empathize with and understand a patient's situation. Doctors are more effective if they can display warmth, genuineness and unconditional regard for their patients.

Roger Neighbour (Neighbour 1987) describes five check points that describe the stages of the consultation.
- Connecting — the connecting of the doctor with the patient's symptoms and signs, ideas and worries
- Summarizing — sharing the doctor's thoughts and ideas with the patient

- Handing over — handing back to the patient information and the degree of self reliance and responsibility to manage themselves.
- Safety netting — sharing with the patient the questions 'What if' or 'What shall we do if' about the symptoms getting worse or the treatment not working.
- House keeping — making sure that the doctor looks after his/her own mental and psychological health in between patients and after a surgery.

Because of the demanding nature of some consultations it is helpful if doctors have sources of professional or personal support. They also need to be aware of wanting to be needed by their patients thereby creating undue dependency. It is for these reasons that methods of obtaining peer group support, receiving constructive feedback on performance, and developing self awareness are so important in enhancing our effectiveness as doctors. It is these methods that will be considered in the rest of this chapter.

How do doctors learn to consult?

Medical students usually enter clinical training with well developed interpersonal skills and are then faced with the demand to collect large volumes of clinical material from patients. They see a role model of a houseman who has to cope with a large number of patients in a limited time. It is not surprising that they want to learn the right questions to ask and how to control the patient who insists on talking about any other worries or concerns. However Byrne and Long (1976) when speculating about the causes of the lack of flexibility they observed, stated that 'Once doctors have developed their style there is a danger that it becomes a prison in which they are forced to work'. This is particularly true of doctor centred styles which close doctors off from any feedback from their patients. One approach to helping practising doctors be more patient centred would be to change teaching and the environment in medical schools. This is beyond the scope of this book, but the pressures that apply to students continue to affect them as doctors during their professional lives.

The most effective teaching programmes have three ingredients: an explicit model of what is to be learnt, opportunities for practice, and feedback on performance. For medical students this is the clinical history, clerking patients, and presentations on ward rounds. However students are rarely asked questions such as 'What is the patient worried about?', 'What does the patient know about their problem?', or 'What does the patient want us to do for them?'. Equally the pressures in general practice may contain these ingredients. These can be the need to stick to time during surgeries, and the approval of the senior partners if you do, and missing the coffee or, worse, being branded as a non-coper if you do not. Patients have a major investment in their doctors and rarely make any negative comments directly to them. However in patients' surveys however the most consistent findings are that they wished that their doctors were able to give them more time and more information during their consultations.

Maintaining the doctor's motivation and enthusiasm depends on a clear sense of direction and regular positive feedback on performance. For this reason it is essential that we have methods of assessing and reviewing things that are important such as effectiveness, and do not confine feedback to those things that are easily measurable such as risk factor recording or prescribing rates.

Possessing a clear framework of what it is we are trying to achieve makes it easier to learn from the example of others, whether this is watching other doctors consult as a student or trainee, or during peer review of the consultations of colleagues as a practising doctor.

Other methods have been found to be effective in developing the doctor's personal attributes. Attitudes can be modified by peer group discussion, and an extended period of structured discussion of cases focusing on the doctors reactions to the patients problems can lead to 'A modified change in personality' (Balint 1957). Inter-personal process recall (IPPR) is a specific training technique developed by Norman Kagan in which doctors are invited to recall what they were thinking or feeling at each stage in a recorded interview (Kagan *et al.* 1963). The aim is to develop the doctor's self awareness and to establish greater control over their feelings.

It is unfortunate that many of the opportunities described, such as working in groups to develop models of effective consulting, reviewing consultations, and discussing attitudes and feelings, are more readily available for general practice trainees and trainers leaving the majority of practitioners relatively isolated. We will now consider ways in which this isolation could be overcome.

CASE STUDIES

The individual doctor

Jerry was a new partner in a long established practice that had been considering training for years but where the partners had been unable to get round to applying. The partners were hoping that he would bring about changes in the practice but gave him limited scope to do so. He was concerned that his consulting skills development which had started in his training practice would cease without anybody to give him feedback or help with his further development.

He already had a structure for analysing consultations and was reasonably clear in his own mind about the difference between an effective and not so effective consultation. Unable to find any other partner within the practice to join him he set about video recording his consultations. He contacted the local VTS course organizer who was able to lend him the PG centre equipment and discuss with him the technicalities of setting it up and obtaining consent of the patients. After a slightly tricky time explaining to the rather conservative staff what he was going to do, he recorded a surgery. He was pleased to notice that most patients were pleased to be involved and thought that it was a very good idea.

He was able to view the consultation at his leisure on his home video recorder when the children had gone to bed. He was pleased to note that in spite of being under time pressure in the consultation he was still able to sit back and listen to the patients without interrupting. He was disturbed to see that the computer on the desk took his attention away from the patients and he resolved to allow time to put all the appropriate information into the computer between seeing patients.

The whole exercise of reviewing his recording consultations only took two hours in the evening, while his wife was at her evening class. Jerry ended his experience with a boost to his confidence about his day to day consulting but with a clear plan about some areas for change. He approached his next few surgeries with interest and a challenge to improve. He also resolved to involve his partner the next time.

The practice: a multidisciplinary approach

The Hamilton Road practice had recently moved into its new premises and the disruption was settling. The practice nurses had sorted out a number of the issues needed to achieve Band 3 Health Promotion and the diabetic clinic and asthma clinic were up and running.

Every two weeks all the doctors, practice and attached nurses got together for their educational meeting with subjects presented by the members as well as visiting speakers. Julie, the practice nurse with a special interest in health promotion, was concerned that the patients were receiving very mixed messages from the doctors and nurses as regards diet and smoking. She said, 'I think that we all agree that these subjects are important and we are consistent in our use of the same leaflets as each other, but still the patients get inconsistent advice. Some of us tell the patients what to do, some give motherly advice, others have a more laissez faire approach and two of us use the "Helping People Change" approach developed by the HEA'.

'What do you suggest we do?' she was asked.

'Why don't we look at our individual approaches and come to some consistent view and then review our consultations in the light of the discussions? Let me offer you a plan' she suggested and wrote on the flip chart.
- Review approaches to effective health promotion in the one to one consultation.
- Agree a suitable approach that all of us can live with.
- Arrange training either from the local primary care facilitator or in house with a distance learning pack.
- Change our way of consulting with patients who need and want life-style change.

- Each of us videotape a surgery including patients who need life style changes.
- Review the consultations in one of these meetings and offer constructive feedback.

'I think that we would learn a lot from this exercise and our patients hopefully would be a healthier lot by the end of it'.

As you might imagine there was a lot of discussion and a lot of 'but what's' and 'what if's' but in the end there was agreement to give it a try. You will not be surprised to hear that Julie was given the job of reviewing approaches together with Derek, the junior partner. They were greatly helped by the local health promotion unit who not only produced the information but offered help in developing their approaches. Between them they developed a training package for the practice of two half days. They used the local amateur dramatic group to play patients so that the doctors and nurses could practice their new found skills.

The two training sessions went off well, they arranged locum cover, and PGEA approval. They negotiated with the FHSA that nurse cover could come out of the training budget. Everyone came but Joe, the senior partner, who had a pressing engagement that meant he missed the role play. Everyone was very pleased with the video review that happened two months after the training sessions. Most had changed their way of consulting. Nearly everyone felt that patients needing help with life style change were now a challenge that they could cope with rather than an issue to avoid.

The receptionist group at their next meeting felt that they too consult with patients and would benefit from developing their communication skills. This was discussed with the practice manager and the doctors and a training day was set up for them. The local amateur dramatic group was enlisted again to play patients with a series of different problems and situations. Each receptionist then dealt with a patient, while being video recorded Afterwards the whole group discussed the consultation using the same criteria and rules that the doctors and nurses used in the previous meeting. These sessions developed the skills of the receptionists as well as giving them a real sense of professionalism and pride in their job

A STEP-BY-STEP GUIDE

The medical press is full of evidence that patients wish to play a more active part in the consultations. As we have seen they have ideas and worries. They have thoughts and wishes about what investigations they should have, and suggestions about possible treatments. People, when ill, often want to do something for themselves, and welcome suggestions from their doctor. These ideas, worries, suggestions, and wishes, might not necessarily be medically correct, but if you seek them out and discuss them with the patients, you can help the patients take a more active part in their consultations. The following steps will help you develop your consulting in a patient-orientated way.

Step 1. Reduce working isolation

Consulting is an individual and personal activity. Few doctors share what goes on in their consulting room with anyone except the patient. If you wish to develop your consulting, it is very much easier to learn together with others of like minds. The other learners could be partners, trainers, young practitioners, members of audit groups, or just a group of friends getting together. There are also many other people in the Primary Health Care Team, who consult with patients and much successful learning can be multi-disciplinary sharing with health visitors, practice nurses, community psychiatric nurses, or any other professionals. You only need one other person with whom to start that process.

Step 2. Decide what you want to achieve in a consultation

This is the starting point of any development process. There are a number of different models, for looking at the consultation, ranging from Balint (1957) to Byrne and Long (1976), from Neighbour (1987) to Cox and Mullholland (1993). The one that we suggest is the one which we described earlier in this chapter. This method is task orientated and consists of the tasks already set out in Table 4.1.

The suggested way forward is to discuss these tasks with the others in your group and agree that you will look at and assess consultations in these terms. As you will see there are a number of values expressed in these tasks e.g. patients have ideas about their health; patients are able to understand their condition; patients have a right to take part in decision making about their own health. These issues need to be discussed and agreed before the next stage is started.

If you are working on your own, think about the tasks, and compare them with your previous ideas of what you were trying to achieve in your consultation.

Step 3. Observe the consultation

When trying to improve, it is important to be as specific as possible, and to think in terms of each consultation rather than consultations in general. To share your consultations with others, you will either have to record it on video or audiotape, or invite direct observation by sitting in. Making a recording of the consultation is easier, more effective, and less disruptive for both doctor and patient, with the added advantage that the consulting doctors can also directly observe the process. Many training practices are using videorecording of consultation in the teaching of their trainees. It has been found that with proper informed consent that the majority of patients are pleased to help their doctors use their consultations to develop consulting skills.

It is important to be aware that the General Medical Council has issued strict guidelines regarding the use of informed consent and doctors should obtain a copy before recording (GMC 1994). They emphasized that true informed consent is obtained from the patient before the video recording is made. Table 4.2 shows an example of one of the consent forms that is in use at Oxford.

Table 4.2

OXFORD UNIVERSITY & REGION
Postgraduate Medical Education and Training
Consent form for videorecording consultations

Dr ...., whom you are seeing today, is videorecording this surgery. The tape may be shown to other doctors for teaching purposes present within the practice* and local doctors teaching courses outside the practice*, only with Dr................. and then it will be erased. Any examination that includes removing clothes or of an intimate nature will not be included in the recording. [* erase if appropriate]

At any time you are free to say that you would rather not be involved in this exercise. If this is what you wish, please let the receptionist know that you would rather not be recorded and the camera will be switched off. If you agree that this consultation can be recorded and then afterwards change your mind, please let the doctor or receptionist know and the tape will be erased.

If you have any questions or there is anything that you do not understand please ask the receptionist.

I understand that my consultation is to be videotaped for teaching doctors and I agree to it.

....

I have had my consultation videorecorded for teaching doctors and I agree to it. being used.
[Sign this after you have seen the doctor]

....
Name ....

Date ....

OXFORD UNIVERSITY & REGION
Postgraduate Medical Education and Training
Video Recording Consultations for Teaching Purposes

This practice is part of the national scheme for developing and training general practitioners. Part of that training involves the very important aspect of effective communication within the consulting room. The purpose of the teaching is to help doctors to become more 'user friendly' to the patients.

To achieve this the doctors need to see themselves consulting and discussing the way they work with other doctors in order that they can find out how they are doing. This is why your doctor today is asking your permission to record this consultation. You will see that the reason for doing this is to look at the behaviour of the doctor rather than at the patient.

If you give permission the tape will only be viewed with your doctor present so that he/she can learn from it. Your doctor will look after the tape as carefully as if it was your medical record and will make sure that it does not fall into the wrong hands. It will be will erased within 1 year.

There are a number of teaching situations locally in which your doctor might be involved where this videotape might be used:

● Teaching within the practice with two or three doctors.
● Teaching at the Postgraduate medical centre at the local hospital with a group of doctors
● On a teaching course with more experienced doctors.

Whatever the circumstances, no-one other than doctors or teachers of doctors will be looking at the tape. If the tape is to be shown to doctors outside the practice you are very welcome to view the tape before you give your permission for it to be used, ask the doctor or receptionist if you wish to do this.

{Cross out those that do not apply to this recording session)

Do feel free to ask your doctor about teaching and learning on the consultation, or any other aspect of this video recording.

Step 4. Compare performance with set objectives

Either on your own, or in the group, the crucial step now is to assess how the consultation you are observing matches up to the ideal which was agreed in Step 2. When setting aside time to review consultations it is crucial to remember that it cannot be rushed. It is also important to have confidentiality and working equipment.

It is necessary to be as objective as possible, and recognize the good points or strengths of the consultation as well as the weaker points which need improvement. We have developed 'rules' for looking at the consultation with others, which make the lessons that can be learnt much more effective. The essential elements are:

- The doctor in question participates first — if you can be honest, you are your own most effective critic. You can see what you wish to change, but it is usually more difficult to recognize those aspects which you have done well. Which is why the next element is:
- Good points first — It is important that you are able to recognize those aspects of your consultations which are effective. It is these aspects which need to be continued. This stage is equally important whether you are on your own or in a group.
- Recommendation not criticism — Each poor point needs to be matched with a recommendation for improvement. An example would be 'I would like to have found out what the patient was worried about, I should have listened more, and not kept interrupting when she was speaking'.

Step 5. Improving the less effective parts of the consultation

By the time you have finished looking at the consultation you should have an idea of a number of things:

- Those parts of your consultation which matched well with the ideal consultation. You will need to continue to develop these good points, and become even more skilful in these areas.
- Areas of the consultation that could have been more effective.
- Recommendations, either from yourself or others, on how you might improve or develop your consultation skills. It is helpful if these aspects can be as specific as possible — for example. 'I think that you are too controlling —' is much less helpful than 'I think that if you listened more, didn't interrupt the patient and helped her to talk more by looking at her, smiling, and making encouraging noises, you would have found out what she was worried about'.

The recommendations can be of different natures. They may be strategic, i.e. suggesting a different course of action. An example is 'Maybe if you considered counselling that anxious patient rather than prescribing, the consultation might have been more effective.' Alternatively the recommendations may be skill based suggesting different ways of how to do things, for instance: 'If you had found out what the patient knew about the subject first, then based your explanation on her knowledge, and then checked out if she had understood it, she would have been more likely to have followed your advice'.

Other diverse issues can arise from observing your consultations. Those may be knowledge of drugs or disease management. Your attitudes to a particular type of patient may be highlighted as may be other beliefs or attitudes. All these aspects can arise out of observing consultations and can be the basis of developing effectiveness.

Step 6. Include the changes into everyday practice.

After Step 5 you will have identified a number of things which you wish to change in your consultations and you will have made a plan of how you are going to do it.

It can be difficult to bring about change in consulting skills. Time is at a premium and patients become very used to our style and method of consultation; they can feel uncomfortable if it is changed. Inclusion of new consulting skills into everyday practice needs careful planning, and you might find the guidelines in Table 4.3 useful.

Table 4.3 Guidelines for new consulting skills

Action	Example
Divide the change planned into small manageable amounts, and do one change at a time. Become comfortable with one new skill before starting another.	Start by asking patients their ideas and concerns with about their symptoms. When that feels comfortable you can start joint decision making.
Make a written plan for yourself at the beginning and the end of each surgery. Mentally review each consultation to see what was achieved.	Plan — this surgery I will check out the understanding of all patients to whom I offer tablets or advice.
Practice new consultation skills at times when there are not so many pressures.	It would be most unwise to try new skills on a Friday night surgery loaded with extra appointments.
Continue to practice a skill until it stops feeling awkward. Change your words until you feel comfortable with them.	If you do not like 'What do do you think is wrong with you'? then try 'Have you any ideas about what might be causing this?' or 'What might have started this off'?
Do not be put off by the patients' initial reaction. It is probably new for them too, and they might need some explanation.	'I was asking because some people might be worried about symptoms like this, and I wondered if you were'.

Step 7. Check out the change by observing again

The final step in developing your consultations is to find out if you have changed. Has the learning process been effective, have you been able to reinforce the message to yourself, and have you been able to maintain the changes? To keep up the momentum of change it is important to review your consultations on a regular basis.

Improving your consultation skills is as important as keeping up to date with medical advances, but it takes time, effort, and persistence.

CONCLUSION

Consulting using this patient centred approach does not necessarily take longer. Initially, as both you and your patients are learning new skills and developing this means of communication, it feels awkward and time needs to be taken. But after a short while time will be saved by the patients being able to tell you their worries more easily, and not needing to consult again with the same problem.

Our experience is that this approach makes patients feel more involved and more satisfied with their consultations, and satisfied patients usually produce a happy and satisfied doctor.

REFERENCES

Arntson, P. (1989). Improving citizens' health competencies. *Health Communication* 1, 29–34.

Balint, M. (1957). *The doctor, his patient and the illness.* Pitman, London.

Buckman, H. and Frankel, R. (1984). The effect of physician behaviour on the collection of data. *Annals of Internal Medicine*, 101, 692–6.

Byrne, P. S. and Long, B. E. L. (1976). *Doctors talking to patients. HMSO*, London.

College of Health (1991). *Ask the patient* College of Health, London.

Cox, J. and Mullholland, H. (1993). An instrument for assessment of videotapes of General Practitioners performance. *British Medical Journal*, 306, 1043–6.

General Medical Council (1994). *Guidance for doctors on videorecordings of consultations between doctors and patients, and other medical procedures for the purposes of training and assessment.* General Medical Council, London.

Greenfield, S., Kaplan, S., and Weare, J. E. (1986). Expanding patient involvement in care; effects on patients outcomes. *Annals of Internal Medicine*, 102, 520–8.

Kagan, N. Krathwohl, D. R., and Miller, R. (1963). Simulated recall in therapy using videotape — a case study. *Journal of Counselling Psychology*, 10(3), 237–43.

Levenstein, J., McKracken, E., McWhinney, I., Stewart, M., and Brown, J. (1986). The patient centred clinical method.1. A model for the doctor–patient interaction in family medicine. *Family Practice*, 3, 24–30.

Ley, P. (1988). *Communicating with patients.* Croom Helm, London.

Neighbour, R. (1987) The Inner Consultation (1987). MTP Press, London.

Pendleton, D., Schofield, T., Tate, P., and Havelock, P. (1984). *The consultation; an approach to learning and teaching*. Oxford University Press.

Pendleton, D. A. and Bochner, S. (1980). The communication of medical information in general practice consultations as a function of patients' social class. *Social Science and Medicine*, **14A**, 669–73.

Podell, R. N. (1975). *Physicians guide to compliance in hypertension*. Merk, USA.

Savage, R. and Armstrong, D. (1990). Effect of a general practitioner's consulting style on patients' satisfaction: a controlled study. *British Medical Journal*, **301**, 968–70.

5 Joint working: learning from experts

Tim Huins

INTRODUCTION

Many educational opportunities occur in everyday general practice, particularly within the consultation, which is the focus of this chapter. It will provide a different slant from most of the other chapters which examine learning outside the consultation. The expert in this context refer to a third party — usually a consultant — who sits in with the general practitioner. The consultants can come from any discipline, but experience has shown that one of the most likely choices is a psychiatrist because of their ability to look at the process of the consultation, as well as the content.

The educational opportunities that exist are often missed due to the pressure of work. However, the more skills that general practitioners acquire, the more consulting will become effective as a result and patient care will benefit. Nor indeed is the general practitioner the only beneficiary. Our consultant colleagues do not have many opportunities to work within primary care and most could benefit from the knowledge and experience that joint consultations in general practice provide.

The complexities and diversities of patient problems presenting in general practice can often defy the specialty centred training that doctors have received. Thus the combined expertise provided by the opportunity to work with someone else provides valuable learning and support. Professional relationships are enhanced also. We all experience anxiety and uncertainty from time to time in consultations, compounded by the pressures of time. Unless this anxiety and uncertainly are resolved, doctors may be affected by self-doubt and patient problems may not be resolved fully.

Referral to consultants or other experts is the usual way of seeking help, but this denies the GP the opportunity to learn together. In the past domiciliary consultations provided such opportunities, but these have now sadly declined in number. Alternatively, a local out-patient consultation at which the patient, general practitioner, and consultant colleague would meet together goes some way to achieving the objectives. These opportunities have become more frequent as fundholding practices have enticed specialists and other professions to their premises.

Out-patient clinics

Rodney Turner (1990) from Thamesmead describes ten consultant clinics held at the health centre since 1980. These clinics had the following aims, which it is appropriate to list:
(a) to resolve diagnostic doubt
(b) to review problems commonly presenting in general practice
(c) to seek advice on management, taking account of any recent advances in treatment
(d) to discuss cases of difficulty, e.g. where the conventional treatment appears to have failed, and where patients are dissatisfied
(e) to improve the standard of referrals and referral letters.
These clinics were in the following specialties:
Paediatrics
Psychiatry
Child psychiatry
Chest medicine
Neurology
Dermatology
General surgery
Orthopaedics
Gynaecology
Rheumatology

With time each of the clinics at Thamesmead evolved differently responding to perceived or changing needs. In the paediatric clinics other members of the heath centre staff, such as health visitors at school and clinic nurses, attended regularly. The rheumatology clinic, including demonstrations of joint and soft tissue injections, resulted in more patients being treated in the practice without referral. The psychiatric clinics were preceded by a working lunch attended by doctors, students, a clinical psychologist, and a community psychiatric nurse. The child psychiatrist, accompanied by his social worker, interviewed the whole family. This was recorded on video and watched in an adjoining room by the family's doctor, health visitor, social worker, and students and sometimes also by a community physician, school nurse, or teacher. Afterwards all those concerned met over lunch to discuss what had been learnt and to plan management. The general practitioners found the fulfillment of the stated aims of the clinics had contributed to improvements in the standard of patient care. The personal contact with consultants was helpful when referring other patients to them in hospital. The clinics were also invaluable for continuing education. This ten-year experience provides a good example of what can be achieved.

Working with psychiatrists

There have been many references, particularly in the field of psychiatry, where the specialist and the general practitioner have worked together. I intend to draw upon these, and from my own experiences working with the late Dr Benn Pomryn, a former consultant psychiatrist at Littlemore Hospital, Oxford. Benn Pomryn worked with many of us in the Thames Valley using the methods I am about to describe.

Almost all general practitioners now accept psychiatry as integral to their work. Minor mental disorders are common in the general population and impose a heavy burden on medical services (Watts *et al.* 1964; Shepherd *et al.* 1966). Robertson confirmed this for the neighbourhood of Aberdeen (Robertson 1979). He stated that if general practitioners did not deal with most minor disorders, psychiatrists would be overwhelmed and would see many patients whose problems did not require their expertise or lay in some other field altogether. This is what happens in countries where the protective shield of general practice is weak and there is direct access to consultants (Horder 1988). Patients consulting general practitioners are more likely to do so with some apparent physical complaint, whether as a manifestation of mental disturbance or as something coincidental and yet linked (Shepherd *et al.* 1981). This is a particular hurdle for doctors starting in practice, struggling to help patients who are reluctant or unable to accept the real origins of their trouble (Horder 1988).

Seminars on psychological problems in general practice pioneered by Balint (1957) were one of the few formal opportunities for psychiatrists and general practitioners to meet jointly to study patients from their respective viewpoints. Lesser and Wakefield, writing in 1975, stated that unless a psychiatrist actually works in a family practice setting it was difficult for him to appreciate the family clinician's unique role. In some respects the family doctor has unique advantages — continuity of care, variable points of contact, and a special rapport with patients. Thus he or she can wait patiently for an opportunity to effect change, a luxury unavailable to the consultant psychiatrist who sees the patient for only one type of problem. Brown and Tower sought the views of general practitioners in one health district by postal questionnaire in 1988. It appeared from the study that about one fifth of general practitioners in S. E. Kent had developed some sort of link with a psychiatrist who worked in their surgeries, but only a small minority of them participated actively in joint decision making. The usual pattern of out-patient clinics does not give general practitioners and psychiatrists the chance to influence each other. Shepherd *et al.* 1981) showed that most consultations for psychiatric or emotional disturbances take place in general practice and few of these are referred to the specialist services. The advantage of joint consulting for patients is that they can meet the specialist accompanied by their general practitioner in familiar surroundings.

Up to now, the National Health Service has provided few opportunities and little encouragement for hospital doctors and general practitioners to work together. But Benn Pomryn writing in the Health Service's Journal in 1983 described how bringing a consultant psychiatrist into the surgery helped GPs to develop consultation techniques, their relationship with patients benefitting as a result. The educational aspects of this three-way consultation (Alexis Brook, *Journal of the RCGP* 1967) makes these observations also.

HOW THE APPROACH CONTRIBUTES TO THE PRACTICE AND WHEN IT SHOULD BE USED

Psychiatric illness in the community

Psychiatrists over the last twenty years have acknowledged that most patients with psychiatric conditions do not come to them. It has been estimated that twenty to twenty-five per cent of all patients seen in general practice consultations have a psychiatric disorder as the only or major problem (Shepherd *et al.* 1966, Goldberg and Blackwell 1970). Since only a fraction of these are referred for specialist care, it has been estimated that general practitioners spend up to a third of their time dealing with psychiatric problems. Carr and Donovan (1992) have queried how resources may best be deployed to deal with all these problems.

The arrangement described in this chapter involves the psychiatrist working in general practice. He or she can also be involved in educating other members of the primary care team. Reception staff are confronted with psychiatrically ill patients, as are district nurses and practice nurses, counsellors, GP trainees, medical students, and social workers. The contribution to the practice can therefore extend through all members of the primary care team, growing with successive contacts with the psychiatrist, not only formally but also informally at such times as the mid-morning coffee break. Community psychiatric nurses and psychologists can also form part of this team.

Meeting the needs of the general practitioner

There are important aspects of the relationship between general practitioner and consultant that need to be fostered and developed. Efforts have to be made to understand the roles of each participant. Mutual respect, trust, and empathy are essential ingredients for success. Ideally the responsibility for the duration and direction of the consultation should rest with the general practitioner and be negotiated carefully. The psychiatrist's approach to the consultation will inevitably need to be modified from the customary model and at times confined to rapid methods of intervention. The general practitioner will have to be prepared to expose his or her inadequacies and to accept constructive feedback.

The teaching and learning tasks can be stated as follows:

1. To diagnose the patient's problems accurately and quickly. The patient's agenda will be the core of the consultation. The consultant brings expertise and the general practitioner prior knowledge of a relationship with the patient, often over many years. The combination will hopefully achieve a satisfactory outcome.
2. To identify each participant's needs. The patient, the general practitioner, and the consultant will have their own needs to be identified during the consultation. The two doctors present will be learning from each other's techniques and at the same time pooling their knowledge and expertise. The patient will hopefully benefit from their knowledge, skills, and attitudes as a result. He or she has the freedom to contribute at any time.
3. To advance participative learning in the primary care setting. This form of learning is a powerful ingredient of effective postgraduate medical education. Joint consultations may take place on several occasions, creating a unique opportunity for learning. This may extend into group activities, either in the practice or with local colleagues. Such a group has met for many years in our local district, resourced in the past by both a psychiatrist and subsequently a psychologist.

Other opportunities

The present changes taking place in the health service could encourage learning from experts. The clinics developed in primary care over the past decade, particularly in asthma and diabetes, would benefit from occasional consultant input to support the work of the practice nurses and general practitioners. In many practices there is already co-operation between doctors and nurses to enable trainee district nurses, health visitor students, and social worker students to sit in with the general practitioners in the consultation and to pool their expertise.

Another obvious example is physiotherapy. A number of practices now employ physiotherapists to work on their premises. Joint consultations between doctor and physiotherapist with individual patients can produce similar benefits to those described for general practitioners and psychiatrists. Other possibilities are chiropodists and dieticians.

CASE STUDIES

The following case studies have been extracted from my records over a number of years and illustrate the kind of benefits that joint consulting brings.

Case study 1 Mr W. F.

My first few years of enthusiastic attempts to keep pace with this patient's multiple symptomatology soon gave way to a sinking helpless feeling each time he appeared to see me. His notes were large and occupied a disproportionate section of the morning's collection of notes. He had been at Dunkirk and fought in North Africa and Italy. These had obviously been his halcyon days. Disappointing employment had followed the twenty years after the war. I imagined him as a shop steward with negative responses to each new innovation. His symptoms seemed to move clockwise round his body. I was unable to help with his problems to either his satisfaction or mine.

One auspicious day, Dr Benn Pomryn was sitting in with me. Mr W. F. was waiting outside the consulting room. I greeted him affably, or so I thought, but Benn detected that Mr W. F. was more disgruntled than usual. When asked why he felt so aggrieved, he responded: 'When Dr Huins calls in his patients he is normally smiling. When he sees me he is not!' This gave us both the unique opportunity to review our relationship, his symptoms, attitudes, and expectations. Time was afforded for me to state how I felt in relation to the situation, with Benn Pomryn facilitating the discussion.

This initial and the subsequent consultations would not have taken place without a third party to highlight the difficult relationship which inevitably develops with some of our patients in general practice. The frequent attender is a potential area for review in these triangular consultations, extended if need be to other members of the family. The outcome in this case was an enhanced relationship between the patient and his GP and a valuable understanding for the years ahead.

Case study 2 Mr and Mrs C.

Mrs C. aged 66 had a blood pressure that I never satisfactorily controlled over 25 years and a number of somatic symptoms that eventually concealed an underlying frustration with her marriage. 'Everything had been fine until the war'. Her husband had been captured in the Far East and spent four years in captivity. 'He returned a different man from the one I married'.

Our consultations were often exciting and animated. I struggled to find satisfactory solutions to her problems. Her husband used to bring her up to the surgery and would stay quietly in the waiting room. I became aware of this with time. Mr C. then began consulting on another day 'Just to have a chat' he would say. He smiled in a particular way when I referred to his wife.

Ultimately after several efforts we coaxed them together, hoping that we could facilitate their relationship after all the post-war years. We witnessed Mrs C. in control of the consultation and Mr C. prepared to spend time 'on the ropes'. Mrs C. did not wish to exchange blows, but hoped to be chased around the ring occasionally, and to have a more exciting relationship with him.

Mr C. watched Mrs C.'s verbal sparring with the two doctors. Interpretations were made and explored. Ultimately we were rewarded with some gratitude and insight into their predicaments and observed some improvement. Without Benn Pomryn's presence I would have had difficulty in venturing into this situation. I benefited from the experience, particularly as the patients' ages corresponded with that of my parents.

Case study 3 Mrs L. D.

Mrs L. D. had mild aortic stenosis. She had been informed of her diagnosis alas a few years before. She spoke about it frequently, centering most of her symptoms in that area of her anatomy. She had helpful and caring children but her husband obviously enjoyed his whisky, sometimes to excess. I too had the impression at times that he could have been driven to it. Mrs L. D. was a quiet, gentle person but never failed to mobilize the junior hospital staff into carrying out more and more investigations on each and every out-patient attendance. Efforts to prise her care back to general practice were met with resistance and her notes grew larger in both locations.

Her 'heart ache' was explored at the regular meetings with Dr Benn Pomryn over several months. He tactfully explored her relationships and fears for the future and I coped with the significance of her mild aortic stenosis and her lack of physical symptoms. Strategies were suggested and the positive aspects of her life explored. A diary was suggested to record the enjoyable parts of each day and the negative portions too. We were not able to involve her spouse, but eventually her heart ache was understood and tolerated and she found some rewards that she was better able to appreciate.

The guidance that Dr Pomryn gave to the patient and to me enabled a chronic attender with a cardiac label to be supported and some aspects of her life enhanced. Her expensive and unrewarding investigations were reduced to a minimum and her confidence correspondingly improved.

Case study 4 Mr and Mrs D.

Mrs D. had presented with several dramatic episodes of anxiety, both at home and in the surgery. Mr D. was invariably out. I had an inkling that this was a clue. Fortunately Mrs D. consulted on a day that Dr Benn Pomryn was present. 'You seem to have a great deal that you are frightened of' he asked. 'My husband always seems to be with attractive females', was the initial response. His job decreed such. However, a description of her first disastrous marriage followed and her equally unhappy and eventful childhood. An avalanche of problems appeared to have been unleashed.

A series of joint consultations followed to explore these problems. They were so diverse and complicated that I would have had some difficulty venturing into these areas alone. Her husband eventually joined us for several sessions, but we seldom found that we could circumvent his inscrutable smile and elusive responses to our discussions. Their daughter eventually provided an invaluable agent for change in the relationship and for improving Mrs D's ability to contain her anxiety and her circumstances at home. Her life became more tranquil and satisfactory as a result.

General themes

These four case studies illustrate the anxiety and uncertainty that both the patient and the general practitioner experience, particularly in prolonged and frequent consultations. The consultant colleague provided the guidance, support, and insight to enable all parties to continue the exploration of unhappy or unsatisfactory situations. These patients did not exhibit severe psychiatric conditions, but are typical of those seen in general practice. Most would probably not have reached out-patient consultations and the option to consult jointly in this way enhanced the therapeutic content and outcome. The GP was able to offer useful information with his background knowledge and this must have accelerated the therapeutic process. Collaborative strategies were planned by all three parties.

The general practitioner was able to use the expertise of his consultant colleague and acquired sufficient confidence and expertise to reduce his out-patient referrals. At the same time the patients received specialist psychiatric help in a familiar, unthreatening, and convenient environment.

STEP-BY-STEP GUIDE FOR THOSE WHO WISH TO USE THE APPROACH

Pre-conditions

The members of the practice should agree the aims and the working method for the joint sessions and identify which doctors wish to participate. The consultant and the receptionists should be present at these discussions, particularly because there are implications for the appointment system. It has been found that 20 minute consultations are about right.

Ethics

Consent is sought verbally on each occasion that the patient attends for the joint consultations. The reception staff welcome patients and tell them that their GP has a colleague consulting with him. Patients have the option of asking to see their GP alone. A hand-out can supplement this information and allows time for patients to reflect and state their preference. A notice in the waiting room is also useful when welcoming patients. The general practitioner has the opportunity to check that they are content for the joint consultation to proceed when welcoming patients into the consulting room.

Our experience is that patients very seldom object to joint consultations, whether they are with consultants or other colleagues in the primary health care team, especially those in training. In fact there have been occasions when the boot was on the other foot. One patient retorted 'I don't mind at all. You are on your best behaviour when you are accompanied!'

Logistics

It should be emphasized that each participant, patient and doctors alike, should be able to contribute freely during the consultation. The positioning of the chairs in the consulting room is important for optimum communication. A triangular format, unemcumbered by a table, helps this process. Additional participants, such as the relatives of the patient or trainee GP, can hopefully be accommodated in the consulting room as well. Examination couches may need to be removed. The consultant should be introduced by the GP as a friend or colleague and by name. His or her discipline may be been mentioned prior to the consultation but it invariably becomes apparent as the consultation progresses.

The consultation process

The consultation should proceed in the usual way. While one doctor is talking with the patient the other monitors progress. If one doctor falters or needs a pause to review the discussion, the other takes over. If things are not clear, the observing doctor can intervene.

Evaluation

It is helpful to record and ultimately to receive feedback on the sessions, both from the consultant and from patients. Possible activities to monitor can include specialist referrals, prescribing, and the subsequent consultations with individual patients. It is also useful to examine the effect on the team as a whole.

Portfolios

Chapter 8 describes the construction of a portfolio for individual learning activities. Joint consultations and the learning resulting from them are obvious examples for inclusion.

CONCLUSION

Many of my colleagues who experienced the joint consultations with Benn Pomryn over a decade ago still remember them with gratitude for the educational and personal support for their patients and for themselves. We hope that his example will encourage other joint consulting ventures to follow.

Horder (1988), has eloquently encapsulated the educational aspects of joint consultations. GPs, especially younger ones, want the specialist to enter into the clinical problems of general practice, especially those that are common, worrying, fascinating and current. This method of working encapsulates principles of learning which are known to be effective. It is immediately relevant to the doctor, helping to solve a problem being tackled at the same time. It is personal, actively involving the learner and it promotes personal and professional development.

Benn Pomryn wrote in 1983:
'Yet, in spite of, perhaps because of, the stresses and pressures assailing GPs, it is impressive to watch those who invite dual consultation. These GPs know a great deal about many of their patients, not only in clinical terms, but also in terms of their everyday lives. With many of these patients the GP has made many attempts to resolve problems with little tuition other than the experience gained and modified by trial and error. He comes to terms with his ability and his desire to help. Some patients show considerable ability to appreciate factors operating for their doctor.'

REFERENCES

Balint, M. (1957). *The doctor, his patients and the illness*. Pitman Medical Publishing, London.

Brook, A. (1967). An experiment in GP/psychiatrist co-operation. *Journal of the Royal College of General Practitioners*, **13**, 127–31.

Brown, L. M. and Tower, J. R. (1990). Psychiatrists in primary care. Would general practitioners welcome them? *British Journal of General Practice*, September (**338**), 369–71.

Carr, V. J. and Donovan, P. (1992). Psychiatry in general practice. *The Medical Journal of Australia*, **156**, 379–82.

Goldberg, D. P. and Blackwell, B. (1970). Psychiatric illness in general practice. *British Medical Journal*, **2**, 437–43.

Horder, J. (1988). Working with general practitioners. *British Journal of Psychiatry*, October **153**, 513–20.

Lesser, A. C. and Wakefield, M. D. (1975). Using the psychiatrist. A different approach to consultation. *Canadian Family Physician*, 79–85.

Mitchell, A. R. K. (1985). Psychiatrists in primary health care settings. *British Journal of Psychiatry*, **147**, 371–9.

Pomryn, B. (1983). A shrink in the surgery. *The Health Services*, 12.8.83.

Robertson, N. C. (1979) Variations in referral patterns to the psychiatric services by general practitioners. *Psychological Medicine*, **9**, 355–64.

Shepherd, M., Cooper, B., Brown, A. C. and Kalton, G. W. (1966). *Psychiatric illness in general practice*. Oxford University Press.

Shepherd, M., Cooper, B., Brown, A. C., Kalton, G. W., and Clare, A. (1981). *Psychiatric illness in general practice* (2nd edn). Oxford University Press.

Turner, R. (1990). Consultant clinics in a health centre. *Update*, **90**(10) 1083–7 (15 May).

Watts, C. A. H., Cawte, E. C., and Kuenssberg, E. V. (1964). Survey of mental illness in general practice. *British Medical Journal*, **2**, 1351–9.

6 Using a facilitator

Peter Havelock

INTRODUCTION

In a *Guardian* leading article of January 1990 Mikhail Gorbachev was described as '*The Great Facilitator: a transitional figure, indispensable to the transformation of the Soviet Union, but not surviving perhaps to see the process completed*'.

Facilitation as a development process has been part of the business and industrial world for some time. In many big companies the training department takes on this role. In others it is taken on by outside experts to help with organizational development, which is one of the functions of management consultants. During the last ten years facilitation has become part of Primary Health Care.

As the dictionary suggests, to facilitate is to make something easier; thus when done properly the facilitator eases the group through the process of solving a problem, making a decision, redefining the goals, or re-stating expectations and responsibilities. Louis B. Hart in his book *The faultless facilitator* (Hart 1992) described key attitudes and behaviours of a facilitator.

- Remain neutral
- Keep the focus
- Be positive
- Encourage participation
- Protect individuals and ideas
- Do not evaluate
- Suggest methods
- Prepare a member to record
- Educate the members
- Co-ordinate

A facilitator is different from a trainer. Trainers define goals for the group Facilitators focus primarily on the process of the group and the needs of the people within that group: the content and direction is decided by the members. The facilitator needs to have different roles at different times. Sometimes he or she will be a passive observer of the process: at other times the facilitator needs to record and feedback process. Yet another role is to add insight and guidance to encourage development. The facilitation of the Strategic Planning Workshops described in Chapter 3 is very much in the non-detective mould.

Facilitation in Primary Health Care takes many forms. There are different models in different parts of the country in various stages of development. Most of it is 'directed facilitation', that is, the facilitator has a personal agenda. This might be to encourage effective prevention, to improve prescribing efficiency, or to establish quality measures. The skills of facilitators working in this way are continually being stretched to maintain the balance between their agendas and those of the practice.

Facilitation began in an ad hoc way in 1981 with Dr Arnold Elliott, supported by the North East Thames RHA, helping Islington GPs improve their premises. This has been described by Judith Allsop in her monograph *Changing primary care: the role of the facilitator* (Allsop 1990). As mentors have worked with individuals, so facilitators have worked with practices (See Chapter 10).

The main driving force for work in primary care came in 1982 from the Oxford Centre for prevention in primary care with the Oxford Model. This focused on the prevention of ischaemic heart disease and stroke. The work has been evaluated showing that considerable change can be achieved by a helpful nurse facilitator guiding the practice (Fullard *et al*. 1984; Fullard *et al*. 1987). Hillary Fender (Fender 1991) described the original concept of the facilitator as focusing on giving practical help and information for setting up systems for risk factor screening and being a 'cross pollinator' of good ideas and practice. The facilitator undertook no service work except to demonstrate skills to staff. The main 'tasks' of the facilitator were:

• to assist team working (setting up meetings with primary care team members)
• to plan and organize prevention and screening activities
• to develop practice nurse skills in health promotion
• to set up a system of medical record audit to measure progress

This model has continued to expand and in January 1994 there were 305 facilitators in post in the UK (Wilson 1994). The majority of them are female with a nursing background: some have additional qualifications in, for example, health visiting or health education but this profile is changing as the role expands. Some facilitators have a specific area of work such as AIDS, computer development, audit, or mental health. But the majority see their role as broader, to include health promotion, team development, staff training, and quality. Whatever the individual subject matter the process of how they work is similar. This is to empower the practices to develop quality health services. They do this by helping the team members to help themselves by providing contacts, information, practical guidance, resources, ideas, training, and co-ordination. The National Facilitator Development Project based at the Churchill Hospital, Oxford, provides training and co-ordination and it can give further information.

In 1991 Medical Audit Advisory Groups were established and a number have chosen to use the facilitator model to achieve their objectives. Nurse and medical audit facilitators have been appointed to help the practices audit and achieve an improvement in the quality of their work. They are often involved in education and staff training and work loosely with the GP tutor and other educators of primary health care teams. Other direct employees of the

FHSA, such as the medical and pharmaceutical advisors, are working in a similar way realizing that this is more effective in bringing about change than either the stick or the carrot approach.

HOW THE APPROACH CONTRIBUTES TO PRACTICE

Diversity and co-ordination

There is a great diversity in UK General Practice. In all the parameters that it is possible to measure the range is enormous. Examples are practice size, members of the primary health care team, referral patterns, amount of chronic care, prescribing costs, and consultation rates. These measures stem from the fact that not only are patients all different, but general practitioners are equally different. Each practice is at a unique stage of development, with individual needs that either help or hinder it to move on. This heterogeneity makes primary care difficult to influence but as Horder *et al.* (1986) said it needs a variety of methods, from a variety of people if we are to produce change. If facilitators are to be successful they must recognize this diversity.

Primary health care is recognized by government and the health authorities as being the main vehicle for delivering effective care to the majority of the population. Because many organizations have a stake in developing this care, the number of people involved can be confusing. Moreover there are occasions when general practitioners are absent from decision making because of their clinical commitments. For this reason facilitators, general practitioners, and other key people need to have a forum within which to meet. These people should include the GP tutor, VTS course organizer, FHSA nurse and medical advisor, MAAG facilitator and others.

In our own locality this group is known as the Wycombe Primary Care Education Forum. It not only uses the expertise of its members to develop individual programmes but also knowledge of the practices to recognize unmet educational needs.

Potential roles

With over 300 in post in Britain and this number expanding, facilitators should be available to most of the primary care teams in one form or another.

Many practices will have very specific needs. Here are some examples of facilitator work:
- organizing study days on diabetes
- supplying records cards for health promotion
- helping practice nurses with asthma audit
- running or managing practice away-days and helping develop a strategic plan

- introducing the practice manager to the local trust training officer
- supplying names of nurses who are looking for practice nurse posts
- helping with information technology
- providing names of other practices who have developed specific protocols
- providing details of where to go for statistical advice
- providing help with patient satisfaction surveys and analysis

Teamwork

Facilitators can perhaps be used most effectively when they address the way in which the practice team works. The importance of teamwork is now generally recognized, as is the fact that general practitioners cannot manage the increasingly complex nature of care on their own.

Facilitators have to recognize that teams are at different stages of development and sophistication: they thus need different types of help and assistance. This is diagrammatically represented in Fig. 6.1.

At a basic level the facilitator can help with developing the practice report and changing this into practice development plans. Alternatively the facilitator can encourage the professional development of practice staff which can take the form of practice nurse education and support groups and the education of receptionists and practice managers. The natural development of this is multidisciplinary education in the form of workshops and study days. These allow members from the same team to learn together and develop action plans in a particular area such as diabetes, access to the practice, or smoking cessation.

Once the team members have started learning together and appreciating the worth of each other the facilitator can introduce opportunities for development:
- making practice meetings more effective
- arranging for the practice to have an away-day for strategic planning
- arranging team workshops, to develop a particular clinical or managerial area
- helping develop research or audit projects or directing the practice to other resources

These activities engender an increased sense of teamwork which can boost further development in a number of different ways.
- Total Quality Management involving all members of staff in the quality of the service provided.
- Assessing population needs and identifying educational and resource requirements.
- Involvement of the community in their own health care, liaising with local groups and organizations.

If they are unable to be of assistance most facilitators are able to point practices in the direction of the information or of someone else who can help.

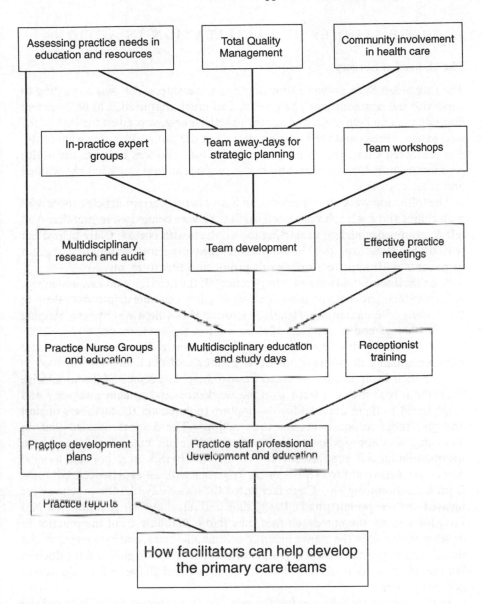

Fig. 6.1

CASE STUDIES OF FACILITATION IN ACTION

The Oakenden Surgery

The Oakenden Surgery was a four doctor partnership which was struggling to cope with the new contract. There seemed so much that needed to be done and limited time and help to do it. Ann, the practice nurse, was given the task of the new patient checks and the well man clinic, but did not really know what to do. She contacted Clare, the primary care facilitator, who was based in the health promotion unit. Clare visited Ann in the practice to find out what she wanted and what her plans were.

The following week she returned with a number of current articles about well man clinics and a selection of record cards that were being used in practice. Ann felt much more confident in starting to run the health checks. Clare helped her with the practical aspects of blood pressure measurements, setting up a register of patients with hypertension, health promotion literature, etc.

Soon the doctors and nurses in the practice felt the need for guidance and advice in helping their patients with lifestyle changes. Clare was able to introduce them to the training officer at the local Health Promotion Unit who was running a 'Helping People Change' course and four of them went to the next session.

The doctors by this time were feeling less pressurized by outside events and were recognizing the value of the other members of the team. They wished to develop their team further and asked Clare to help. She came and discussed with them the possibility of a team working workshop and a team away-day and emphasized to them the need for the doctors to empower the members of staff and give them responsibility for their actions. The doctors decided that an away-day was appropriate to their stage of development. Clare was able to negotiate financial support for this from the FHSA and booked a local conference centre at preferential rates. Together with an experienced GP tutor from a neighbouring area Clare facilitated the away-day. All the practice were pleased, the receptionists had a lovely time and felt that their point of view had been listened to; the nurses felt that they had a mandate from the practice to develop their role in the management of asthma, diabetes, and hypertension; the practice manager had a team of people who had a common goal and the doctors felt that the practice really had plans for the future and all the staff would help in achieving them.

In time the practice did not feel the need for their contact with Clare and she moved on to help another practice.

The Wycombe Primary Care Prevention Project

When the WPCPP started, we had the same initial aims as the Oxford Project: to encourage the identification of risk factors in the local population for coronary heart disease and to audit the primary care records to monitor progress in increasing coronary health. In the Health District there are 207 doctors in 37 practices. Within the first two and a half years of the project, the facilitator visited 34 of the practices, audited 26 of the practices' records for prevention data (smoking, blood pressure, etc.), and helped set up screening clinics in 24 practices. We achieved the initial aims of the project in the majority of the practices within three years.

We were also aware of many other changes occurring within primary care during this time. We observed an increase in Primary Health Care Team Meetings. (Many practices did not meet as a team before 1986.) The use of a Structured Record Card for recording risk factors, which encourages the reorganization of the practice records, became more prevalent. All the practices, except one, had installed a computer by 1990, recording their list of patients, demographic details, risk factors, therapy, and major disease episodes aided by working closely with Wycombe Primary Care Computing (a local computer support group).

The number of practice nurses in England and Wales trebled between 1985 and 1991. A local practice nurse group was started in 1986 for mutual support and education. Interpractice visiting of doctors and staff also increased, decreasing their isolation and permitting the exchange of ideas and data. Increased attendance at educational study days for skill development was also noted. The study days were mostly organized for the whole team, rather than for one professional group. In this way, teamwork was emphasized in conducting health promotion efforts in the local community.

Practices started to look at their practice populations, as having identifiable groups of people with specific needs. The improvement in the record systems enabled them to identify groups according to age, health habits, disease, family history, circumstance, treatment, and more recently, area/housing.

Thus the doctors and the primary health care teams have moved from the identification of risk factors in an individual to the identification of needs within the community. This required different skills. Educational sessions met those needs. From 1986 to 1991, the following sessions were conducted for primary care providers; in 1986 — smoking, nutrition and obesity, and hypertension; in 1987 — looking after yourself and prevention by teamwork; in 1988 — handling people and paper, communication skills, and time management; in 1989 — Asians and coronary heart disease and patient education in diabetes; in 1990 — assessing need, promoting health in the Asian population, and total quality management. The subject matter gradually changed from medical issues to more process- and team-oriented issues.

Knowledge about individual conditions was supplemented by handouts, guidelines, or protocols, but the skills had to be learned, practised, and developed. Across all of the educational sessions, providers' attitudes and communication skills for effective health promotion were constantly reinforced, regardless of subject matter.

USING A FACILITATOR — A STEP-BY-STEP GUIDE

These steps are set out in a logical order but in certain circumstances a different order may seem more appropriate.

Stage I — Establishing the need

This is probably the most important aspect of practice development with a facilitator
- Recognizing the need for help
- Being in a frame of mind to ask for help

When feeling under great pressure it is difficult to allow oneself the time to stand back and realize that something can be done about the stresses of daily life. Anyone in the practice, doctor, nurse, practice manager, or health visitor can come to this realization and start the difficult process of convincing the others of the need for help.

Stage II — Discussion within the practice

For the practice to be able to accept help from the facilitator it is important that a significant number of the 'opinion leaders' (often the doctors and practice manager) accept the need for change and development. It is then vital that they are able to convince the others that outside help is the answer to some of their problems and obtain agreement to proceed.

Stage III — Discovering local resources

There will be a number of people in the locality who will be aware of sources of help and facilitation. This list below contains examples but should not be regarded as comprehensive. The FHSA is frequently able to help and funds many facilitators.
- FHSA — staff training officer
- Health promotion unit staff
- Medical Audit Advisory Group members
- GP tutor
- Postgraduate centre staff
- FHSA nurse advisor/medical advisor

Nationally: The National Facilitator Development Project,
              Churchill Hospital, Oxford, OX3 7LJ.   Tel. no: 01865-226035

Stage IV — Seting up the initial meeting

The need for proper planning has been stressed. The facilitator will need briefing about the practice, what the initial needs are, and what is expected of her. It is

helpful for the practice to have a contact person that makes sure the arrangements are finalized. The timing of the meeting will need to suit the key players
and an adequate length allowed.

Stage V — What then?

Plans made at the initial meeting should be renewed regularly and it helps
considerably to involve the facilitator. This makes it more likely that they will be
achieved: the facilitator can respond if the practice needs help. The practice
needs to identify what further resources are needed. These might be special
expertise or skills, staff time, specific training, record cards or information
booklets or computer skills. The facilitator, or someone she knows, might well
be able to help: part of her job is to build up a wide range of local contacts. She
can provide support and encouragement to specific members of staff who wish
to develop their roles. Examples are: a nurse setting up an asthma clinic; a
receptionist wanting to do a patient satisfaction survey; a health visitor wanting
to do a presentation. The facilitator can monitor developments with the practice
member and guide everyone through difficult times.

Stage VI — Further developments

Once the practice has achieved its initial plans and found the benefit of the
facilitator it is time to take stock. The facilitator can often help the practice to
develop in ways discussed in other parts of this book. Some of these might be:
● Further training
> In house
> Courses both locally and further afield
● Quality improvement projects
● National Conferences for Primary Health Care Teams i.e. The ACT con-
ference
● Team development workshops
● Practice team away-days
● Multidisciplinary study days
● Research projects — contact with the local university
● Becoming involved in teaching — of medical students, nurses, trainees, or
receptionists

IN CONCLUSION

Asking a facilitator into the practice can have a major influence on that
practice's development. It does more than achieve change; it will help to
develop team working within the practice. This relieves some of the burden
on the doctors, as they share their vision for the practice and feel that everyone
is working towards it.

REFERENCES

Allsop, Judith (1990). *Changing primary care: the role of the primary care facilitator*. Kings Fund Centre, London.

Fender, H. (1991). Facilitators in primary health care. Who are they, and what are they doing? M.Sc. Dissertation Department of General Practice, Nottingham University.

Fullard, E., Fowler, G., and Gray, J. A. M. (1984). Facilitating prevention in primary care. *British Medical Journal*, **289**, 1585–7.

Fullard, E., Fowler, G., Gray, J. A. M. (1987). Promoting prevention in primary care. Controlled trial of a low cost, low technology approach. *British Medical Journal*, (1994). **294**, 1080–2.

Hart, Louis B. (1992). *The faultless facilitator*. Kogan Page, London.

Horder, J., Bosanquet, N., and Stocking, B. (1986) Ways of influencing the behaviour of general practitioners. *Journal of the Royal College of General Practitioners*, **36**, 517–21.

Wilson, A. (1994). *Changing practices in primary care: a facilitators handbook*' Health Education Authority, London.

7 Peer review through practice visits

John Hasler

INTRODUCTION

During the first 30 years of the British National Health Service, general practitioners were coming to grips with defining the discipline of primary medical care. We have touched briefly on some of the features of that development in Chapter 1. 'The Future General Practitioner' (RCGP 1972) was one of the earliest attempts to map out the work of the modern general practitioner. The MRCGP Examination was by then rapidly attracting an increasing number of candidates and through this, experienced general practitioners were starting to make judgements about standards of care.

By the end of the seventies the Royal College of General Practitioners decided to see if it was possible to move the assessment of doctors into their practices. The Board of Censors set up a Working Party in 1980 to test this hypothesis and those of us involved in that exercise decided to call our report 'What sort of doctor?' (RCGP 1981).

It goes without saying that our first task was to attempt to identify the hallmarks of a competent and caring family doctor. We had between us wide experience of general practice and aspects of its development. But we found that adopting criteria from previous publications proved somewhat problematical. So we decided to return to first principles and use our common sense to agree what it was patients expected of their doctors. This was devised in the first instance without any thought of whether these attributes could be assessed. And although the original aim had been to produce primarily an assessment method, the results had as much influence on education and its development. A second working party examined the possible uses of the methodology. It concluded, amongst other things, that it embodied the principles of peer review and that both assessed and assessors realized that they were taking part in mutual learning and research (RCGP 1985).

THE CONTRIBUTION TO PRACTICE

In this section I shall review the original criteria and subsequent features of visiting: I shall look at its use in Oxford region training practice assessments and our experience over a decade.

Criteria

In the first working part, we eventually decided on four broad areas of performance (RCGP 1981).

These were:
- Professional values
- Accessibility
- Clinical competence
- Ability to communicate

All except the first were fairly obvious attributes. However when we came to consider these three we concluded that there was something missing — something that we came to call professional values. Under each heading was a list of sub-headings and the full list can be found in *'What sort of doctor?'* (RCGP 1985).

We also needed to come to some conclusion about acceptable behaviour under each subheading. For this we produced criteria set out as paired statements indicating the good and bad extremes. For example under home visits, the statements read:

GOOD	BAD
'The doctor is prepared to visit patients in their homes: clear arrangements exist for requests'	The doctor is very reluctant to do home visits: arrangements for requests are confusing and difficult for patients'

and under prescribing:

'His use of drugs is appropriate He has a disciplined and logical approach'	'The use of drugs is inappropriate He gives no evidence of a disciplined approach'

The Oxford experience

At Oxford we produced a rather similar list of headings for the development of priority objectives for vocational training (Oxford Region Course Organizers and Regional Advisers Group 1988).

These were:
- Patient care
- Communication
- Organization
- Professional values
- Personal and professional growth

There were a number of sub-headings in each section. They were selected as priorities because we considered them crucial, commonly required, both now and in the future, and generalizable: that is to say once learned in one situation, they could be used in other situations.

In the early eighties, some of the thinking behind the '*What sort of doctor?*' approach was used in the development of new criteria for the appointment of trainers at Oxford: these criteria remain relatively unchanged today (Schofield and Hasler 1984).

For example:

'The trainer should display a high standard of clinical competence in his or her consultations, the long term care of patients, preventative medicine, prescribing, record keeping, auditing his or her work, and appropriate use of other members of the practice health care team and of colleagues in agencies outside.'

It was clear from the outset of all these developments, that there was significant overlap between the individual doctor's activities and those of the partners and team. Indeed modern high quality primary health care depends as much on the work of nurses, managers, and their staff as it does on doctors, so the Oxford training practice criteria includes, for example:

'The practice must be committed to reviewing and auditing the care it provides for its patients. The partners and other members of the health team should be able to demonstrate how they identify strengths and weaknesses in the care of patients and how they take appropriate action to improve that care'.

Consulting the assessed

The more detailed the criteria became and the more that they may be used in some kind of assessment that might have sanctions attached, the more important it becomes to make sure that the criteria are acceptable to the assessed as well as the assessors. In the original development of Oxford trainer criteria, a working party which included a representative of every trainers' group devised the list and trainers are consulted before modifications are made.

Criteria for practice visiting, then, need to be explicit and acceptable to both parties. They will inevitably relate to the other members of the practice as well as to the individual doctor.

Methodology

Once criteria have been developed it is necessary to produce a systematic plan by which their achievement can be assessed. In the original '*What sort of doctor?*' working party, we eventually selected six sources of information from which we could reach conclusions (RCGP 1981).

These were

- The practice profile (pre-visit questionnaire)
- Direct observation of the practice and its functioning
- Discussion with staff and partners
- Inspection of records and registers
- Review of videotaped consultations
- Interview with the doctor

Each of these activities produces material which can be used to assess one or more of the criteria. In the original college field trials the criteria were largely considered appropriate, the method was acceptable, and the sources of information generally valuable. Reliability was generally good. The main difficulty related to the assessment of clinical competence, self-awareness, and personal behaviour (RCGP 1985).

Participants agreed on the potential value of the exercise as an educational experience although some were disappointed that the feedback was not as critical as they thought it might have been.

From a strictly educational standpoint the development of visits has not been as widespread as it might have been hoped. This is probably because of the time and effort involved and because of the tendency, referred to above, of doctors to be insufficiently hard-nosed when it comes to criticizing colleagues. Where the method has been adopted as the basis for training practice approval visits, (as at Oxford) considerable experience has now been acquired.

Sources of information

The six sources of information have remained largely unchanged although the practice is asked to audit its own records in advance which enables a much larger number to be scrutinized. It also has the advantage of those being assessed to see the strengths and weaknesses at first hand. Records are also selected on the day, some of which relate to specific problems so that it is possible to audit the practices' own protocols, for example, for the management of asthma or depression.

The visitors

There is no doubt that the visitors gain considerable benefit from the visit. The arrangements for Oxford training practice visits specify that all trainers and course organizers are visitors, although not on their own patch. This means that the visits are indeed largely peer review.

Because the quality of care depends not only upon the doctors but also on the way the practice is organized and run, we now include a practice manager in the visiting team. This has extended significantly the range of comments available for the practice into such areas as health and safety at work, the way decisions are made, and the responsibilities of employers. The use of practice managers is currently being evaluated.

Having four visitors affords the opportunity for them to divide up and conduct more than one interview simultaneously. The doctor is always interviewed by all the doctors but not the practice manager who does not view videotaped consultations. However it also means that time has to be found during the day for the team to share information and cross check what each member has learned.

Feedback

After such a detailed assessment those being visited feel anxious about what has been unearthed. Therefore it is important that some feedback is given at the end of the day. The person in charge of the visit must have the necessary skills to do this and at Oxford we emphasize the need to follow a set procedure which is based on that described in the assessment of consultations (Pendleton *et al.* 1984). These are briefly that good points are listed first and that areas for consideration are described in the form of recommendations for change.

It is important to realize that the majority of practices in the UK never receive detailed feedback about their performance except in very crude terms such as grateful letters or complaints. Our experience leads us to conclude that a detailed assessment of a doctor's activities by a peer is one of the most potent and relevant forms of education.

Reports

After the completion of a training practice visit a report is compiled on an 18 page standardized layout which helps to ensure that no major areas are missed. The section on management is now usually compiled by the practice manager. The final pages consist of conclusions — the highlights followed by the recommendations.

It is important that these reflect what was said at the end of the visit otherwise there may be confusion. It is also helpful to restrict the recommendations to what needs tackling: it is not appropriate usually to tell the practice how to solve the problem since those working there are likely to be much more adept at understanding the issues.

Conclusion

The development of practice visits, albeit largely confined to training practice assessments, has enabled a large group of general practitioners to become experienced and comfortable with a very powerful learning exercise.

CASE STUDIES

The following studies are based on real visits although the circumstances have been altered. In each case, one item has been highlighted.

Strategic planners

Meadowside was a practice of five doctors with a list of 10 000 patients in a suburban part of a large town. The premises had been built in the seventies and space was at a premium. There were three attached health visitors, three district nurses, and three practice nurses. The practice manager had been appointed in the previous year: before her arrival the doctors had largely taken the management decisions themselves.

The practice was well thought of locally and the standard of medicine was high. Record keeping was good and the doctors and nurses had set up an asthma clinic and started to audit their work. The workload was moderately onerous.

The visitors spent the morning seeing various groups on their own. When they came together at the end of the morning a pattern began to emerge. The doctors were justifiably proud of what they had achieved and the good working relationship within the practice. They had produced a variety of protocols including ones for hypertension and asthma. They met with the practice nurses and manager regularly and saw the district nurses and health visitors two or three times a week over coffee.

The practice nurses were very complimentary about the doctors. 'They will always come if we want something'. The attached nursing staff echoed these sentiments. 'The doctors will always see us between patients if we have a problem'. However the visitors sensed there were some difficulties and some tactful questioning elicited some further information. The protocols for hypertension and asthma had been devised by the doctors on their own and then handed to the nurses to implement. The latter could have pointed out some difficulties if they had been involved from the outset. The health visitors were somewhat jealous of the regular meeting between the doctors and practice nurses: they would like to have been involved as well but had felt it inappropriate to say anything.

The practice manager had found that the partners were experiencing some difficulties in delegating decision making. Nor was she clear where the practice was heading in the next few years.

At the feedback session the visitors were able to compliment the doctors and the rest of the practice on the good relationships and happy atmosphere. They were then able to raise the issue of needing to involve everyone at the outset when protocols and plans were drawn up. They also suggested that the doctors and practice manager sit down together and review what each wanted of the other. A few weeks later the visitors learned that the practice was planning its first away-day in which all the practice and attached staff would be involved. The nurses and managers had been asked to make presentations to help chart the aims for the practice for the next three years.

Protocols and paper

The Greenbank practice consisted of three doctors and various attached and employed nurses in a small village. At the beginning of the visit they proudly presented their protocol book which one of the doctors and practice nurses had spent one year compiling. Altogether some 10 conditions had been tackled including several chronic diseases and a number of common problems. The protocols were well referenced and reflected current scientific thinking. They were extremely comprehensive — the one on hypertension ran to six pages.

The visitors asked to see the records of 20 patients with diabetes. One of the visitors went through these and noticed a number of things. First, it was quite difficult to obtain information on the diabetic care because it was buried in the routine clinical notes. Then she saw that whilst the recording of blood glucose was good there was hardly any recording of feet examination and entries relating to eye examination were rather sporadic. The visitors discussed these findings with the partners after coffee. They complimented the partner who wrote the protocols on how comprehensive and well referenced they were. Then they asked how they had worked out in practice. After a moment's hesitation, one of the other partners said she found them difficult to use. They were rather long and she could not remember all the details. She had also noticed that it was difficult to know how well they were doing because the relevant information was hard to locate. The visitors and partners talked about this for a while. The third partner wondered if flow sheets would help and the visitors encouraged the partners to try them. A few weeks later the visit leader received a letter saying that introducing diabetic flow sheets had not only reminded the doctors and nurses what they had to do but had highlighted some major deficits in their care. Everyone had come to realize that while the protocols had made everyone feel good, on their own they had had little effect on the quality of the practice work.

Ideas and concerns

The visitors were looking at a videotaped consultation which had been recorded by the training partner. It concerned a rather anxious young woman who had come back for the result of a high vaginal swab taken at a previous consultation for vaginal discharge. The doctor explained that the swab was negative and therefore there was nothing for the patient to be concerned about. The patient responded by expressing anxiety about the discharge. The doctor reinforced the message of a negative swab and the patient left looking somewhat dissatisfied.

The visitors and trainer discussed the tape. The former complimented the latter on his clinical thoroughness and they asked why he thought the patient appeared dissatisfied. The conversation moved on to look at possible strategies in the consultation that might have resolved the issue. One of the visitors asked the trainer what other questions he could have asked. A number of possibilities came up. 'You still look very concerned: why is that?' Or, 'What do you worry about when you notice a discharge?' Or, 'The fact that the swab is negative still leaves you with the discharge, doesn't it? Is that a problem?'

By the end of the session, the trainer had a number of extra questions that he could add to his repertoire that might open up new areas of the consultation and reduce the likelihood of poor communication.

Conclusion

These case studies illustrate a number of general points.
- learning is powerful when it is based directly on one's clinical practice
- feedback needs to commence with good points
- it is helpful if the visited can generate some of the solutions themselves
- collecting information from more than one source often produces a picture which is different to the initial one.

A STEP-BY-STEP GUIDE

Whilst practice visits have been a great success in educational terms they are not activities to be undertaken lightly. They require meticulous preparation and a clear understanding on both sides of what is to be attempted and achieved. We refer to the preparatory discussion where these issues are discussed and agreed as contracting.

The following check lists should enable you to conduct and receive successful visits.
1. What is the purpose of the visit? Both visitor and visited should agree in advance of what is to be done and what will be covered.
   - Are certain areas no-go or is everything to be looked at?
   - Are there specific activities the practice would like studying?
   - Why is a visit being requested?
2. Who will be seen? Is the visit to be restricted to one doctor or will others be seen? Possibilities are:
   - other partners
   - practice nurses
   - health visitors and district nurses
   - practice manager
   - administrative staff
   - others
3. What aspects of the practice will be looked at? Possibilities are:
   - Medical records
   - Computer screens and data
   - Audit reports
   - Appointments book
   - Videotaped consultations
   - Library
   - Medical equipment

4. What data will be supplied in advance of the visit? It is important that certain documents can be studied in advance to save time on the day: it also enables the visitors to pinpoint possible areas of concern. Possibilities are:
   - Practice brochure
   - Audit reports
   - Annual report
   - PACT data
   - Protocols
   - Special audits carried out for the visit, such as a records audit
5. Who will visit? Will it just be confined to one or more doctors or will it include nurses or practice managers?
6. How will feedback be given? Will it be verbal or written or both? Does the person leading the visit understand the rules of feedback with good points first and then specific recommendations?

Once all these things have been agreed it is useful if they are all embodied in a letter in advance so that there are no misunderstandings.

CONCLUSIONS

Visits are a very powerful way of providing feedback to a practice. They are immediate and relevant. There are three major points to recognize:
- Criteria need to be defined first. Unless both parties are agreed about these, confusion will result. If there are no criteria then it is difficult to come to any meaningful conclusions and much of the potential is lost.
- The primary purpose of peer visits is diagnosis. It is about feeding back to the practice and individuals what they are doing well and where there are matters that need tackling. The aim is not to tell people what to do although some ideas can be offered if requested.
- The procedure, if conducted skillfully, can ensure that the practice gets the maximum benefit and that the threats are minimized. People can take any number of suggestions on board if they feel that they have some strong points and they are made to feel valued.

REFERENCES

Oxford Region Course Organizers and Regional Advisers Group (1988). Priority objectives for general practice vocational training. (2nd edn). RCGP Occasional Paper.

Pendleton, D. A., Schofield, T. P. C., Tate, P. H. L., and Havelock, P. B. (1984). *The consultation — an approach to learning and teaching*. Oxford University Press.

Royal College of General Practitioners (1972). *The future general practitioner: learning and teaching*. BMJ Publications, London.

Royal College of General Practitioners (1981). What sort of doctor? *Journal of the Royal College of General Practitioners*, **31**, 698–702.
Royal College of General Practitioners (1985). What sort of doctor? Occasional.Paper, 23. RCGP, London
Schofield, T. P. C. and Hasler, J. C. (1984). Approval of trainers and training practices in the Oxford Region. *British Medical Journal*, **288**, 538–40, 614–18, 688–9.

8 Portfolio-based learning

Roger Pietroni and Lesley Millard

INTRODUCTION

The origins of portfolio-based learning are rooted in experiential learning and embrace the theories of adult education, emphasizing the importance of reflection in learning. The term experiential learning sometimes causes confusion and may mean different things to different people. Some have argued that all learning is experiential. The converse, that all things experiential lead to learning is certainly not true. It is necessary to reflect and process experience for learning to occur. In many areas of medical education, we have often confused educational input with learning outcomes. Time spent or attendance at learning activities has been assumed to mean learning acquired.

Experiential learning involves a sequence of stages at the core of which is reflection. The significance of reflection in learning was highlighted sixty years ago by John Dewey who emphasized the importance of 'reflective activity'. Experience, he felt led to growth and maturity and education. He recognized two forms of experiential processes which led to learning. One process involved trial and error experimentations which would lead to rule of thumb decisions. This process was considered of limited value to a learner. The second process he identified as reflective activity. Reflective activity allowed for effective problem solving to occur. This, Dewey felt would lead to more effective learning. He was one of the first educationists to describe learning as a cycle where reflection continually moved cyclically, back and forth between the experience and the relationships being inferred (Bond *et al.* 1985).

Freire (1972) also emphasizes the importance of reflection to the learning process and his work is relevant. He designed experiential situations which enabled learners to reflect on their understanding of themselves and act accordingly. This combination of reflection in action, he called praxis. Kolb and Fry (1973) developed a model of experiential learning where learning is conceived as a circular four stage cycle. Immediate concrete experience is the basis for observation and reflection, these observations are assimilated into concepts, and a theory from which new implications for action involving active experimentation can be deduced.

Again, reflection is at the centre of Kolb's model. Reflection is seen as an important human activity differentiating man from other animals, where man is able to recapture and process his experience, reflect upon it, evaluate it, and act appropriately. Anything which encourages the association between the experience and the reflective activity which follows it will enable and enhance learning.

We are unlikely to make the most of experience if we are exposed to one new event after another without an opportunity for reflection to occur (Bond *et al.* 1985).

Two useful ways of stimulating reflection are debriefing and keeping a diary or log of experiences. Portfolio-based learning is one such model which incorporates both debriefing (through the use of mentors) and keeping a log (through the portfolio).

The term portfolio is borrowed from the graphic arts. It is a collection of evidence of the learner's experience and achievements during a period of educational activity. Learning can often be spontaneous and elusive. The learner may gain a sudden insight into a problem, a flash of inspiration, an intuitive understanding. Unless this is captured, through reflection, and recorded in the portfolio it may be lost. The portfolio may contain anything that can demonstrate the learning. For example, notes, handouts, papers that have been read, analysis of activities completed, and, most importantly, reflections about the work. Other examples might include videos, audits or projects, case descriptions or commentaries on reading, and log diaries (see Fig. 8.1).

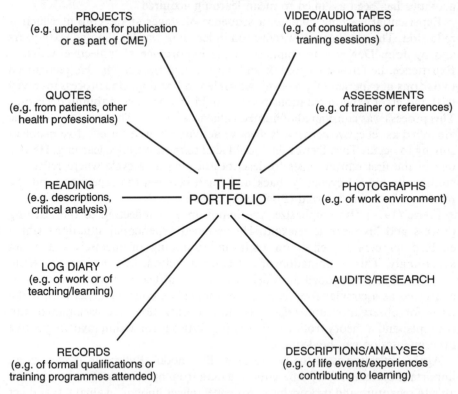

Fig. 8.1 Examples of materials which might be included in the portfolio to demonstrate learning achieved.

Whilst the portfolio itself is a collection of evidence demonstrating the achievements of the learner, portfolio-based learning is a process which the learner undertakes. The portfolio approach allows learning to be centred on the individual learner's needs. It encourages self-directed learning by empowering the learner to assume responsibility for his or her learning. It also offers a wide range of learning opportunities and learning methods which are chosen to fit learning styles and preferences.

A mentor facilitates the whole process by offering the learner a combination of support and challenge. In learning we all need help at times. The idea of having a mentor during health care training received prominence first in the USA and two writers went as far as to say that 'everyone who makes it has a mentor' (Collins and Scott 1988). Mentors are not new. The word mentor dates back to Greek mythology. Mentor was a 'wise and trusted guide' who, for twenty years, had the task of counselling and befriending Odysseus' son whilst Odysseus was fighting in the Trojan Wars. There are numerous mentoring relationships in history. Freud and Jung, Beethoven and Haydn, de Beauvoir and Sartre.

A mentor helps the learner to identify his or her own educational needs and professional development. The mentor is not a teacher but a facilitator who encourages the learner to develop their own strategies and discover their own solutions. She has a key role in helping the learner reflect critically on experience and explore different perspectives. Above all the mentor needs to be able to offer the learner 'unconditional positive regard' (Rogers 1983). That is, to adopt a non-judgemental stance, in which the learner is always valued and accepted.

There is much confusion about the role of the mentor and what it entails. Levinson *et al.* (1978) suggests that the concept of a mentor includes being a teacher, sponsor, counsellor, developer of skills and intellect, a host, guide and exemplar, and someone who can support and facilitate the realization of the mentee's dream his life's vision. This places a huge burden on the mentor and suggests much wider boundaries than are necessary for mentoring within portfolio-based learning. The tasks of the mentor have been identified as offering time and commitment, facilitation, emphasizing strengths, building confidence, advising on timing for moving-on, acting as a sounding board, etc. In the context of portfolio-based learning, the mentor role is more of a facilitator than a teacher, more of a coach than a trainer. The skills are those that are necessary to facilitate reflection, develop self-awareness, help in debriefing, and form an educational plan or learning contract.

In portfolio-based learning, the mentor may help the learner to debrief on a learning experience. To be useful debriefing needs to be structured and follow a sequence. Gibbs (1988) suggests that the stages of a structured debrief follow the stages of the experiential learning cycle and include:

- *Description*: A description of the experience without any judgements or conclusions.

- *Feelings*: A recognition of the feelings/reactions without analysis.
- *Evaluation*: What was good or bad about the experience.
- *Analysis*: Making sense of the experience.
- *Conclusions*: What can be concluded in both general and specific terms from the experience and analysis.
- *Personal action plans*: Making the most of what has been learnt.

Educational plans or learning contracts (Knowles 1986) are set by the learner with the help of the mentor after the learning needs have been diagnosed. They should include details of learning objectives, learning resources and strategies, together with an indication of how the learning will be accomplished and assessed.

Since 1984, portfolio-based learning (Bond *et al.* 1985; Redman and Rogers 1988) has been introduced successfully into various areas of adult learning. One of the early applications of portfolio-based learning was in youth and community work. There was growing concern that while youth and community workers were experienced and were making a valuable contribution, some of them felt the lack of formally recognized qualifications. Portfolio-based learning allowed them to document their achievements and their learning. Their experience and skills could therefore be validated or accredited. APL (Accreditation of Prior Learning) attempts to make more use of existing human resources by ensuring that learners are not taught what they already know and that their experience is recognized and validated thereby allowing a wider access to work and to higher education. The process of APL (Simosko 1991) is based on the recognition that practitioners learn not only by formal methods of education but also at work and in other areas of their lives. Such learning may be of equal relevance to that which is acquired in schools and institutions of further and higher education.

Like the educational plan, the portfolio can be seen as both a product and a process (Bond 1988). The portfolio-based learning process enables the learner to assume responsibility for their own personal and professional development. It encourages autonomy by giving learners major responsibility for planning, managing, and evaluating the learning and allows flexibility in that they can work to their own preferred pace and style. It recognizes the learner's strengths and learning needs. Focusing on the portfolio as a product may detract from its value for enhancing self direction and autonomy.

In recent years, portfolio-based learning has found a place in medical education (Royal College of General Practitioners 1993), not only in continuing medical education but also in undergraduate and vocational training and in a variety of Masters courses.

WHAT PORTFOLIO-BASED LEARNING CAN CONTRIBUTE TO THE PROFESSIONAL DEVELOPMENT OF GENERAL PRACTITIONERS

Demands on the time and energy of general practitioners have increased greatly since the introduction of the recent NHS reforms. There are growing requirements from Government for undergraduate and postgraduate education to demonstrate its effectiveness and relevance to the workplace (Barnett 1992 and Pollett 1987). These two sets of pressures mean that the education of general practitioners needs to be related to clearly identified educational goals, to be seen to have an effect on practice (in both the general and specific senses of the term), and to be viewed by GPs as something which can be fitted into their lives and which will be of positive value to them. Portfolio-based learning offers one way of fulfilling these requirements. The contribution which it can make to the professional development of general practitioners is examined below.

Firstly, portfolio-based learning enables GPs to focus on their experiences. These may be personal life experiences or experiences related to work. The artificial division between learning and life/work experiences which attending courses may foster, is therefore dissolved. Furthermore, the problem of transferring learning from a course back into the work situation is avoided, as learning is built on reflection of work experiences. Identification of specific changes in behaviour may be required as part of the portfolio-based learning process as described on p. 91. Learning and work become interwoven, rather than apparently separate experiences and can be anchored to the everyday achievements, problems, and concerns of the GP.

Secondly, portfolio-based learning enables the individual GP to tailor her learning programme to her learning style and needs rather than accepting off-the-peg educational provision. With the help of a mentor, to ensure that the process is rigorous and well-focused, the GP has the chance to engage in learning which meets the precise needs which she identifies at a time and in a manner which she feels is appropriate. She can make choices which accommodate her learning style and the practical constraints under which she is working. For example, having identified a need to acquire more skills in giving feedback within the practice team, one GP might choose to attend a course entailing a good deal of skill practice. Another, might choose to undertake some reading and use this to identify some specific ways in which to change her behaviour. Both might then attempt to use their learning at the next team meeting, in addition to reflecting, recording, and producing evidence of what was achieved for their portfolio.

Since portfolio-based learning specifies a process, but not a method of learning, as well as accommodating a range of learning styles, it can embrace varied learning needs, requiring different sorts of educational experiences. Examples might be:

- the need for clinical knowledge, such as information about the potential and applications of a new drug;
- managerial needs such as skills of team building and needs related to interpersonal skills,
- attitudes such as those required for working with the families of terminally ill children.

Portfolio-based learning offers the possibility of meeting such diverse needs in ways which are appropriate and accessible to the individual undertaking the learning. As the example above indicates, it does not preclude attendance at courses or other 'ready-made' provision. What it does specify is that the starting point for selection of the means to meet learning needs is the learner, rather than what is on offer in any given educational programme. In this way, portfolio-based learning offers a learner-centred approach, where the learner selects what is suitable to meet her needs, rather than seeking to fit into what is offered. When reading, discussing with colleagues, attending a lecture, or whatever she has elected to do, she has a clear idea of what she hopes to gain, why she has chosen this method of learning, and will reflect on and evaluate what was actually learned. The emphasis is thus moved from attendance to a reflective consideration of the value of the learning which has been achieved.

Portfolio-based learning reflects other tenets of adult education as well as 'starting where the learner is' (Weil and Gill 1989). The learner (with the help of the mentor) is encouraged to celebrate her strengths as well as to identify areas which require further development. While the mentor offers support and challenge, the responsibility for the learning remains with the learner. Her autonomy and ability to determine her own educational pathway is respected (Boydell 1976). This latter point indicates an important link between the approach which portfolio-based learning can encourage and the philosophy of patient-centred doctoring. Just as the GP seeks to understand and work with the patient's agenda, so the person engaged in portfolio-based learning, is helped to identify her own agenda and to work with this. A person-centred approach to identification and clarification of issues and planning of appropriate action, are features of both portfolio-based learning and patient-centred consultations.

While the above discussion refers to qualified GPs, the points made also apply to trainees (Royal College of General Practitioners). A portfolio-based learning approach, with the trainer or another experienced GP to act as a mentor, provides a means whereby the trainee can focus on the learning achieved in day-to-day contacts with patients and the members of the practice team. It can provide a structure for managing learning needs which may otherwise feel overwhelming or chaotic.

The process of keeping a portfolio encourages self-directed learning; an important objective in vocational training. A trainee portfolio may, for example, contain videos recorded at different stages thereby potentially demonstrating skills acquired; audits and projects; notes on papers or books read and trainee log diaries — an important learning tool in vocational training encouraging critical reflection.

In a trainer–trainee relationship there is, of course an unavoidable inequality of experience and power. The process of portfolio-based learning and the tenets on which it rests, are an aid to enabling trainees to assume responsibility for their own learning and to build habits of reflection and analysis which are appropriate to life-long and self-directed study. Similarly, the trainer can view portfolio-based learning as a way of ensuring that a desire to help, to encourage, to teach, does not lead to a didactic or paternalistic approach, which although may be comfortable for both parties, would, in the long run, create patterns of dependency detrimental to effective learning.

CASE STUDIES — EXPLORATION OF PORTFOLIO-BASED LEARNING IN A GENERAL PRACTICE SETTING

In addition to giving some actual examples of the use of portfolio-based learning in general practice on subsequent pages, the longer description here offers a picture of the process, using two fictitious characters to provide a case study. This offers a way of highlighting some of the areas which require consideration when portfolio-based learning is used by GPs. Although the actual scenario is constructed, its elements are drawn from life: the process issues explored, come from actual experiences of people using portfolio-based learning.

Portfolio-based learning using co-mentoring

Dr G. has worked as a principal at a practice in a busy market town for ten years. He is committed to the concept of continuing medical education, but for some time the courses he has attended and his reading have left him with a feeling of dissatisfaction. He usually finds things to interest him in his educational activities and yet they lack sufficient focus. The local GP Tutor invited him to a meeting to hear about portfolio-based learning. This left him interested in the concept but not entirely sure what it would entail. His appetite was sufficiently whetted for him to attend a further session related to portfolio-based learning and the role of the mentor within this. As a result, Dr G. has decided that portfolio-based learning may provide him with a means of identifying and meeting his educational needs and that it may be more satisfying than the 'What's on offer?' approach he has adopted so far. He particularly wants an educational programme which fits both his needs and interests and the time which he has available to study. He hopes that portfolio-based learning will offer a flexible approach and yet will have sufficient structure to help him to follow the goals he sets himself.

After some discussion, he and a principal from a rural practice about 12 miles away, Dr A., agree to co-mentor. In a preliminary meeting, they discuss ground rules and boundaries and fix three further dates on which to meet. They decide that the first meeting will be used to identify learning needs and to begin to explore ways of meeting these. Each will work on their needs between the first and the second meeting; the latter will be a 'How's it going?' session, which will celebrate progress, examine any areas of difficulty, and aid reflection on learning achieved and how it can be utilized. They decide that the final meeting will focus on what needs have been met and the perceived value of the portfolio-based learning process. In addition, each will bring his portfolio to the last session, to give his mentor a chance to see how the learning has been recorded. The GPs decide that the format which will suit them, is to meet at Dr A.'s home, since he can ensure they will have a quiet room in which to work with no interruptions; they will have 10 minutes to settle to the task and remind themselves of their ground rules and then each will have 1 hour of the other's undivided attention, with a short break for coffee in between. They decide to spend 20 minutes at the end reviewing the process. Dr A. remarks that this is a similar set-up to the one his wife uses for co-counselling.

Dr A. comes to the first session with detailed notes and has clearly given a lot of thought to his perceived needs. Dr G. feels somewhat daunted by this and wonders if he has a role, but after a short while he is able to question, reflect back, challenge, and summarize, in a way that helps Dr A. to check whether he has identified needs (areas which relate to important goals he is trying to achieve) or wants (areas which he would like to pursue but are less relevant to what he is seeking to accomplish). Dr A. remarks 'Well, somehow I must get to feel that what I need to do is also what I want to do, or where's my motivation to do it?' This provides the substance of a useful discussion.

When it comes to Dr G.'s turn, he is a bit embarrassed that he has not been able to sort out what he might work on. He explains that he seems to have been going round and round and getting nowhere. 'This is ridiculous; I feel I should know what I need to learn about. I've got lots of ideas, but they don't seem to amount to anything . . .' Dr A. listens and seems sympathetic; Dr G. feels slightly less foolish but still baffled. Dr A. suggests Dr G. puts the problem of what he should learn on one side and suggests that instead Dr G. talks about what he is achieving in his work. Dr G. begins hesitantly but relaxes a bit as he gets going. Some issues arise as he talks and Dr A. draws his attention to these by echoing key phrases and using open questions. By the end of his hour, Dr G. has established that the area he needs and wants (!) to work on is related to HIV-positive patients. He has not identified specific goals, but feels he will be able to achieve this clarification on his own. He can hardly believe that he has used a whole hour in getting to this point. However, he feels confident that the area he has chosen is the right one for him at present.

In reviewing the process, each doctor says what went well and what went less well for him and writes a few personal notes about skills he used and/or felt he required and things to remember for next time. Before parting, they remind one another that observing strict confidentiality is vital.

In the second meeting, Dr A. reports on a half-day course he has attended and time spent in the University library pursing references on heart sounds and diagnosis which was his chosen area. He has written notes on the information has gained, but feels he will not really know whether he has increased his diagnostic skill until a suitable patient appears. He comments that he is surprised by the difficulty he has in analysing his learning, as opposed to saying what material he, or a lecturer, covered.

Dr G. is feeling enthusiastic about portfolio-based learning. He has visited a local hospice, has been in touch with the Terence Higgins Trust, and has read some of the first-hand accounts of people dying of AIDS. He has two HIV-positive patients and feels that the learning he has achieved has been of great benefit in his work with them. He has analysed his last two consultations with these patients and brought some quotes which help to demonstrate how his attitudes have changed and how this change is reflected in his manner. He has included in his portfolio a short poem about a young man who discovers he is HIV-positive. Dr G.'s reactions to this poem are also recorded in his portfolio, together with an account of how he links the poem to his understanding of his patients.

For Dr A. the most important part of this second session is sharing his doubts about what he is achieving and having his confidence and his motivation boosted by his mentor. For Dr G. the important part of the session is identifying his next steps, so the he can build on his success so far.

The third session occurs at the end of six months. The two GPs use it to review their progress, look at each other's portfolios, and to help one another toward a critical evaluation of what has been achieved. Both have found that the process of portfolio-based learning was a demanding one and required a good deal of self-discipline. This they welcomed and also found difficult. They feel that they have experienced an educational process which had been worthwhile in terms of its contribution to their work as GPs and its contribution to their understanding of themselves as learners. Keeping going at times when there was a good deal happening in the practice or in their personal lives, has been hard. Both are surprised at the variety of materials which make up the portfolios. There are written analyses, tapes of consultations, photographs, a poem, a letter sent by a patient, and notes of reading undertaken and lectures attended. Each doctor has a huge sense of achievement and also a feeling of sadness that, at least temporarily, the process has reached an end.

Portfolio-based learning used in a region

In the North Thames (West) Region, a small project was set up to help young principals with the problems associated with the early years of starting in general practice. The first stage involved identifying suitable mentors. In the

North Thames (West) Region, a two year Higher Professional Education Course for young principals has been run consecutively since 1987. It seemed that the graduates of this course would be ideal recruits as mentors. Not only were they aware of the potential problems young principals face, but they had also undertaken a communication skills course as part of the course they had completed. Twelve GP mentors were identified and a one-day training course was set up. The course involved a review of portfolio-based learning and an examination of the skills required to be a mentor. Training exercises involving role play were employed. The skills required of a mentor were identified as:

- providing support
- helping the learner identify their strengths
- helping the learner identify their needs
- helping the learner set educational plans
- encouraging and facilitating reflection
- using responding skills such as non-verbal skills, active listening, appropriate reinforcement, use of challenge, use of reflection, and self disclosure

Six GPs with less than five years of experience in general practice volunteered to embark on a portfolio approach to personal and professional development. They were self selected, keen to pursue a programme of continuing education that was flexible, catered for their needs, and involved them in learning activities that suited their own learning style. They were given short biographies on the twelve GP mentors. From these twelve, the young principals choose a mentor. The choice was made after an initial meeting to ensure mutual compatibility. There then followed a number of stages to the project involving a series of meetings.

The first stage involved a further meeting between GP and mentor to identify educational needs. This would typically begin with an initial assessment of strengths and existing skills and experience. The next stage involved the GP learner (with guidance from the mentor) setting up a learning contract or educational plan. The learning contract stated what the GP intended to do, how she would engage in the learning activity, and what she hoped to achieve at the end of the learning programme and how it might be assessed.

The learner then engaged in the learning activity and kept a portfolio. The portfolio contained anything that documented the learning. Keeping a journal or a log diary was encouraged. The learner was then given an opportunity to practise her newly acquired learning. During this process the learner receives PGEA accreditation on submission of her learning plan. The mentor received PGEA accreditation for the sessions spent with the learner as it was recognized that mentoring is a learning process for the mentor as well as the learner.

The educational plans submitted by the young principals all seemed ambitious with broad objectives which were not clearly focused. The educational plans were however, never intended to be static documents but could be revisited at any stage and modified accordingly. Many of the learning needs identified reflected the recent changes in the NHS e.g. fundholding and administration. The journals or log diaries seemed to be used like educational plans. They logged day-to-day learning needs and ways in which the learner might address those needs. They were also used to log newly acquired learning or to reinforce existing knowledge. The journals were often the focus of discussion with the mentors.

How to use it — steps involved in process

The portfolio learning process begins with the learner identifying and describing an experience. This experience may arise not only from work but also from personal life. Personal life experiences need to be given the recognition they deserve and the learning from these experiences should not be considered of less relevance or less value, than those experiences arising from professional work. Where portfolio-based learning is seen as part of CME, it is, of course, important that the experience chosen has direct bearing on the learner's professional role as a GP.

Learners may be unsure of how to choose an experience to describe. If so, the use of critical incidents or case analysis may prove helpful techniques. Alternatively, learners may be encouraged to describe aspects of their work which give them satisfaction and which indicate areas of well developed skills. From here, they will often move naturally to reflect on areas which they feel they need to develop.

The chosen experience is described to a mentor who facilitates the process by active listening with both verbal and non verbal encouragement. It is important for the experience to be fully described and explored and the urge to draw premature conclusions must be avoided.

After the description, the learner is encouraged to reflect on the experience and to try to identify what learning occurred. The mentor facilitates this process by clarifying, summarizing, and reflecting back to the learner. The mentor may challenge in a supportive manner, to help the learner to a deeper level of analysis, or to elucidate areas which may appear to be avoided. No interpretation is made by the mentor. Following this the learner, with the help of the mentor, looks at ways to go forward by identifying new learning needs and devising an educational plan to meet these needs. As indicated in the scenario of Doctors A. and G., the mentor offers support and challenge to enable the learner to identify important needs, i.e. those which are of significance to continuous professional development. Educational plans or learning contracts are then set by the learner with the help of the mentor. They should include details of learning objectives, learning resources and strategies, together with an indication of how the learning will be accomplished and assessed. Figure 8.2 gives a pictorial representation of the process.

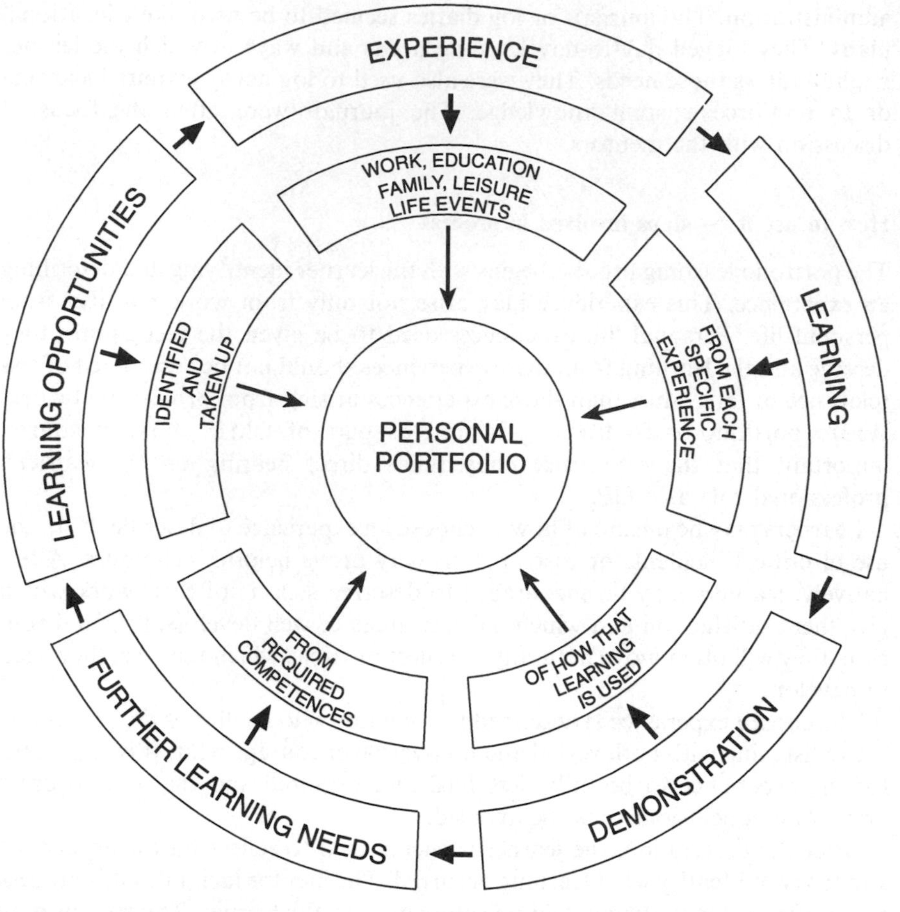

Fig. 8.2 The portfolio-based learning process.

The quality of the process should be evaluated by the learner, as part of the learning cycle. Initial criteria for evaluation should be set when the learning plan or contract is established. These criteria will need to be revisited and revised as the learner gains a deeper understanding of the needs s/he is seeking to meet. Some questions which may be helpful in setting criteria are:

- How will I know when I have met my learning objectives?
- What is it about these objectives which makes me see them as important?
- What reasons can I offer (myself and others) for the choices I have made in order to meet my learning needs?

Some criteria may also be set by external bodies if they are providing accreditation. In all cases, the mentor has a key role in helping the learner to set rigorous criteria for assessment and evaluation. The quality of portfolio-based learning can be judged in two ways: in terms of the type of criteria set by the learner and in terms of the outcomes of the learning. Whether the portfolio is externally accredited or not, the rigorous self-assessment and evaluation of process and outcomes which the mentor can facilitate, is essential for the learner's sense of achievement and the development of the professional skills of self-assessment and evaluation of learning.

It is important to recognize that externally imposed accreditation may affect the process of portfolio-based learning and in consequence the end product. This will be especially true if the accrediting body seeks to dictate content and standards, thus constraining the choice of areas for study and denying the learner a role in selecting criteria by which the work is to be judged.

REFERENCES

Barnett, R. (ed.) (1992). *Learning to effect*. SRHE & Open University Press.
Boud, D. (1988). *Developing student autonomy in learning* (2nd edn). Kogan Page, London.
Boud, D., Keogh, R., and Walker, D. (eds) (1985). *Reflection: turning experience into learning*. Kogan Page, London.
Boydell, T. (1976). *Experiential learning*. Sheffield City Polytechnic, Manchester. Monograph 5.
Collins, E. G. C. and Scott, P. (1988) Everyone who makes it has a mentor. *Harvard Business Review*, July/August 89–101.
Dewey, J. (1993). *How we think*. D. C. Heath, Boston.
Friere, P. (1972). *Pedagogy of the oppressed* (translated by M. B. Ramer). Penguin, Harmondsworth.
Gibbs, G. (1988). *Learning by doing: A guide to teaching and learning methods*. Further Education Unit, Elizabeth House, York Road, London SW1 7PH.
Knowles, M. S. (1986). *Using learning contracts*. Josey-Bass, San Francisco.
Kolb, D. and Fry, R. (1975). *Towards an applied theory of experiential learning*. In *Theories of group processes*. C. L. Cooper (ed) Wiley, London.
Levinson, D., Darro, C. N., Kline, E. B., Levinson, M. H., and McKee, B. (1978) *The seasons of a man's life*. Ballantine Books, New York. 1978.
Pollitt, C. (1987). *Measuring university performance: never mind the quality, never mind the width? Higher Education Quarterly*, Vol 44, No 1
Redman, W. and Rogers, A. (1988). *Show what you know: a workpack for youth and community workers*. National Youth Bureau, Leicester.
Rogers, C. (1983) *Freedom to learn for the eighties*. Charles E. Merrill, Columbus, Ohio.
Royal College of General Practitioners (1993). *Report of a working group on Higher Professional Education. Portfolio-based learning in general practice*. Occasional Paper 63. Royal College of General Practitioners, London.
Simosko, S. (1991). *APL: a practical guide for professionals*. Kogan Page, London.
Weil, S. W. and McGill, I. (eds) (1989). *Making sense of experiential learning*. Society for Research into Higher Education & Open University Press, Milton Keynes.

9 Quality improvement

Martin Lawrence

INTRODUCTION

The pattern of scientific advance is step-wise. A series of separate and apparently disjointed findings seem to imply a chaotic and unstructured world, and then a single unifying theory explains and encompasses them all. Then further findings imply further disorder, until another simplifying theory is established. Galileo provided a framework for understanding the movement of celestial bodies, Nils Bohr gave us a structure for understanding atomic particles. On a more mundane level, quality improvement theory (Total Quality Management suitable adapted for primary care) can do the same for practice and professional development in primary care.

And how we need such a unifying and directing force, for currently we are in real chaos! For over twenty years now primary care has been steadily improving. Initiatives released by the working conditions put in place by the 1966 Charter (BMA 1965) have been multitudinous and diverse, but together with enablement has come obligation. As John Bain described we have become a 'should do' profession, with 'circulars, reports, occasional papers and discussion documents accumulating in the in-tray all subscribing to what general practitioners should do' (Bain 1986). 'What sort of doctor' has instructed us that we must improve in the areas of professional values and communication, as well as of clinical competence and access. (RCGP 1985) We must offer comprehensive acute, preventive, and chronic care. We must manage our practices to ensure access, continuity, and efficiency. We must work with other disciplines and with secondary care. We must base our processes on the best available evidence. But how do we approach the right areas, how do we put our energies into the most suitable area, and how do we know that we are getting anywhere? The proposed solutions have been to increase continuing medical education and to develop practice evaluation or audit.

Continuing Medical Education and its problems

The right to CME was embedded in the 1966 Charter (BMA 1965). Prior to this time most education for general practitioners was conducted by hospital specialists, but the provision of both finance and protected time encouraged the development of postgraduate education devised by general practitioners for general practitioners. Perhaps the greatest evidence of advance was in the development of courses for vocational trainees, which culminated in compulsory vocational training in 1981. Vocational training has a well developed and well funded support structure with regional advisors, course organizers, and trainers, who have both devised and directed the education in order to ensure its relevance. The management and direction of postgraduate education for general practitioners on the other hand has never been adequately financed or structured. The method has been that those who run courses decide what they would like to teach, and professionals attend courses that interest them. At first there was some obligation to attend a certain number of courses a year and expenses were covered: later the obligation was removed but the expenses allowance for those who attended courses retained. Since the 1990 GP contract expenses have been removed, and now the incentive is that a part of general practitioners' income (the so-called 'education allowance') is not paid unless evidence is given of having attended courses (Department of Health and Welsh Office 1989). There is some attempt to encourage a wider scope of education by insisting on a balance of service management, prevention and disease management, but on the whole there is no way of guiding doctors to the educational events that they need. And since the incentive to spend on their education is reduced by removing expenses allowances, GPs tend to attend the cheapest options to satisfy their requirements.

Until now the huge preponderance of effort by postgraduate advisors has been in the area of vocational training, that brief three years before thirty years of practice. The appointment of a network of general practitioner tutors will tilt the balance a little towards continuing education, but unless there is some way of guiding general practitioners' needs to relevant courses a great deal of effort will remain wasted.

As for the rest of the primary health care team — what of their education? Practice nurses' courses remain skeletal compared to those for community nursing staff. Education for clerical staff is unsystematic and usually superficial. No one has responsibility for providing education for either group, so provision varies from district to district depending on who has decided to take up the responsibility — for example it may be a local university department or in the case of clerical staff very often the local Medical Audit Advisory Group. Once again, whether the education is directed to need is open to question; and the whole exercise depends on the general practitioners — the employers — both agreeing and paying.

Audit and its problems

Audit in primary care began in the 1970s and has been one of the growth areas of the past fifteen years. It began by individual professionals becoming involved in peer review, and the Royal College of General Practitioners has been a major influence in its development. The Birmingham research unit of the Royal College of General Practitioners was one of the first units to facilitate the collection of comparative data between doctors and practices with feedback and discussion (Crombie and Fleming 1988); and '*What sort of doctor*', was a landmark in setting standards and criteria against which doctors could review themselves and their practice performance (RCGP 1983*a*). Perhaps the most important development was the RCGP's Quality Initiative which stated (RCGP 1985*b*):

1. Each general practitioner should describe his current work and should be able to say what services his practice provides for patients.
2. Each general practitioner should define specific objectives for the care of patients and should monitor the extent to which these objectives are met.

Gradually audit became more and more integrated into professional practice as professionals realized that they needed to review their work in order to improve their services, and that they needed to be accountable both to their responsible authorities and to their patients.

The history, techniques, and application of audit is comprehensively reviewed in Lawrence and Schofield (1993) — but the technique is best summarized in the diagram of the Audit Cycle developed in that book.

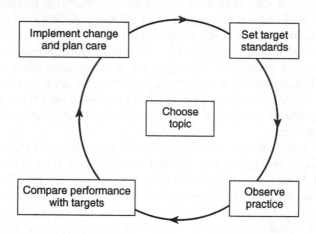

Fig. 9.1

This diagram emphasizes some of the main benefits of audit — that participants have to identify the standards that they are aiming at: they then need to measure their performance to see if they are reaching those standards; and then they must consider what to change to get better.

This exercise if carried through develops professional attitudes in two ways. Firstly by reviewing their performance, both in relation to the performance of their peers and their own target standards, professionals become more realistic about their attainments and so are directed to improve their competence in handling the topic in question as well as their practice in implementation. Secondly, it does direct the educational development of professionals, since the very procedure of being challenged to set standards directs attention to the topic in question, challenging professionals to improve their own competence as well as to seek elsewhere for guidelines to adapt and implement.

There are many examples of service improvement using audit, both in the book quoted above and elsewhere, and few would contend that quality of care improves in relation to the topic reviewed, while professional development is effective for those who take part in the process (Lawrence and Schofield 1993; Humphrey and Hughes 1992). And there's the rub. Work done by the Oxfordshire MAAG shows that in Oxfordshire, probably one of the most fortunate areas for primary care, where 80% of practices are now doing audits which involve setting targets and planning care, only a small range of topics are covered and only a few of the primary health care team are involved (Lawrence *et al.* 1994). So how comprehensive is the professional development, and how much change can really occur?

The response of Government

Up to 1990 in the United Kingdom professional development was exclusively in the hands of professionals. In the new contract (Department of Health and Welsh Office 1989) Government decided to take a firm hand in attempting to improve quality, in two ways. Firstly it decided not only to guide strategy but also to direct the details of some clinical care, by imposing large numbers of targets which had to be attained, either as a term of service or because a large part of income depended on their attainment. This approach is recognized to be detrimental to the attainment of the highest quality of care, because as soon as professionals are set external targets those targets become the thresholds at which they aim. In addition it is the opposite of professional development; development was arrested and doctors expected to aim for the external targets set. They are distracted from areas where they feel that improvements are required, because all too much energy is spent in dealing with the areas that are compulsory. In the event, it has proved to be particularly counterproductive since the areas chosen have corresponded to the accepted values of the mid-1980s (universal health checks), while evidence is moving professionals to an approach more targeted on patients 'at risk'.

Secondly the GP contract placed great emphasis on audit, setting up MAAGs to encourage audit amongst general practitioners (Department of Health 1990). This has tended to over emphasize the place of audit in the provision of quality care, except in cases where MAAGs have had the vision to develop their role. The recognized need for teamwork has led for calls to 'clinical' or 'multi-disciplinary' as opposed to 'medical' audit. But if you put the cart before the horse it lacks direction even if the cart is multidisciplinary. Before audit can truly be effective the service must be satisfactorily planned.

Finally Government also gave Health Authorities the obligation to improve primary health care services in their districts. Here movement has been gradual as authorities have developed their new management role, and they too have been constrained by having to implement external directives. But if Family Health Service Authorities are given increasing freedom and flexibility, then the working together of professionals and managers in an agreed quality improvement programme holds great prospects for service and professional development in the coming years.

In summary, continuing education and audit have failed to provide satisfactory practice or professional development because:

● Continuing education is targeted neither on the needs of the professional nor on the needs of the patients for services. It is determined largely by cost, accessibility, or the interest of the recipient.

● Audit is retrospective and topic based. The topics largely depend on data the practice finds conveniently available, or items decided by Government, often unsupported by evidence.

● Dissipation of professionals' energies into these channels is currently distracting them from a more organized form of practice development, which would provide better opportunity both for improved professional development and patient services.

QUALITY IMPROVEMENT FOR PRACTICE AND PROFESSIONAL DEVELOPMENT

Adopting and adapting total quality management for primary care

We seek a system for professional development which can embrace the best of the continuing education, performance review/audit, and service development which we have already achieved. Such a system is Total Quality Management, developed for industrial quality improvement — but ideal for application to health services, if suitably adapted.

After the Second World War, in the Western world, quality assurance in industry was based on inspection. Goods coming off the end of the line were inspected with two aims: firstly to ensure that not more than a certain percentage fell below a set standard, and secondly to reject, and possibly repair, as many as possible of those of unacceptable quality. It has been called the 'theory of bad apples' (Berwick 1989).

This is rather like medical audit — set a standard, check whether you come up to that standard, if you do (however marginally) breath a sigh of relief, if you do not then review the working practices.

As a method for improving quality this is flawed for several reasons. Firstly, it is a retrospective exercise working on the basis of seeing what has gone wrong and carrying out remedial activity, while looking back into the system to see why the defects have been produced. It starts from the present position and tries to improve it for the future. Secondly, it does nothing to drive improvement for all those areas where performance comes above the threshold, however marginally. Since most products are above threshold, there is no mechanism for improving the quality of most of the activity being examined. Finally, even with remedial action, the only aim is to get the bad apples just the other side of the threshold — not a particularly good aim for an organization trying to attain the highest quality.

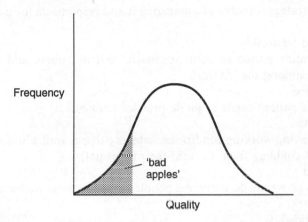

Fig. 9.2

This type of quality assurance by retrospective inspection was questioned by several quality experts, notably Edward Deming, whose theories largely turned Japanese industry from shoddy to high quality output over twenty years (Deming 1986). The new management method depended on looking at every stage of a process, involving everyone working on the process, and developing the best working method at every stage, so that the eventual apples are all good — 'right first time'. At each stage any defect in production is worked on and improved 'every defect is a treasure' — and the process goes on all the time — 'every worker has two jobs, to do the job and to think how the job could be done better'.

Many of the methodologies need adapting for health care because they were developed in industry, where outcome is more easily assessed both numerically and statistically, and where success is more easily measured, in financial profits. The methodology has been adapted for health care especially by Donald Berwick's group at the Institute of Health Care Improvement in Boston, and presented in their course 'Improving Health Care Quality'. Much of their work relates to American health care with its profits motive, and to hospitals — but the systems are highly relevant to our situation also.

Aspects of TQM

Berwick and his colleagues emphasize certain aspects of quality improvement — adapted from Deming's famous fourteen points. The 'new organization' must be:

- focused on quality

    In primary care, do we have a group in the practice dedicated to quality improvement strategy, capable of organizing it and responsible for it against a timetable?
- with committed leadership

    Are the partners united in their approach, and are nurse and clerical representatives among the leaders?
- customer minded

    Do we assess patient needs to guide practice changes?
- employee minded

    Are we improving working conditions, listening to our staff's information and views, and enabling them to fulfil their potential?
- process minded

    When things go wrong do we blame people, or the systems we have set up for them to work?
- statistically minded

    Do we measure activity before and after change to identify problems and confirm their improvement?
- dedicated to continuous improvement

    Do we have a continuous strategy, constantly adapted to need. Or is our audit intermittent and topic based?
- treating suppliers as partners

    How closely do we co-operate with secondary care, social service, or drug wholesalers — or do we get them to compete with each other?
- Innovative

    Do we patch up present systems, or do we have vision in achieving improvement?
- Proactive

    Are we happy to stay good, or determined to be best?

This list comprises a blueprint for professional development, and in many ways reflects a great deal of the teamwork development exercises that many practices have been undertaking over the past four years. But whereas 'teamwork development' can be rather an abstract exercise, and planning exercises often neglect implementation, the use of TQM methods in developing general practitioner performance enables these activities to be focused on practical activity — and raises morale by showing change.

The quality framework

The key model for quality improvement as developed by Berwick is shown in Fig. 9.3, although I have adapted his model for British primary care. It is I believe the most useful conceptual framework for practice development, and hence professional development, that is currently available.

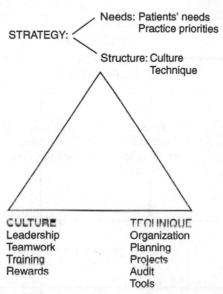

STRATEGY:
Needs: Patients' needs
Practice priorities

Structure: Culture
Technique

CULTURE
Leadership
Teamwork
Training
Rewards

TECHNIQUE
Organization
Planning
Projects
Audit
Tools

Fig. 9.3 Framework for quality improvement in primary care. Adapted with permission from the syllabus 'Improving health care quality'. Copyrighted by the National Development Project.

Firstly it emphasizes that there must be leadership within the practice. TQM may seem to imply that everyone works all the time to improve quality, but unless leaders define strategy nothing can really progress. This is a major advance from audit, or from meeting external targets, because whereas audit can be carried out by a few enthusiasts within the practice, a practice strategy can only be set if the leaders are of one mind. Once the leaders have defined a strategy then all the partners must at least endorse the direction and effort, even if the implementation is delegated to others. The leaders should include leaders of each discipline in the practice, so multidisciplinary working automatically takes place without making special provision.

As relationships between professionals and health authorities develop it is at the level of strategy that there can be negotiation between practices (as suppliers of primary care) and authorities (as the purchasers). It gives an opportunity for the role of authorities in strategic guidance and support to merge with the role of the professions in practice development.

Secondly the model shows that strategy must respond to practice needs and priorities and equally to the needs of patients. The practices' provision of care must no longer be determined by the partners irrespective of the wishes and needs of their patients.

The quality practice

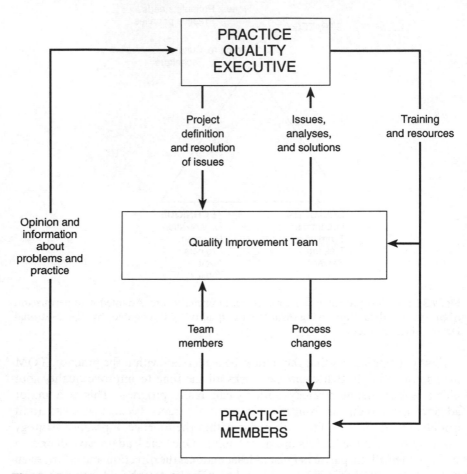

Fig. 9.4 Practice organization for quality improvement.

Thirdly it shows that the practice plan needs two areas to be covered in order to enable implementation; it needs the right culture, and it needs certain skills and techniques. Perhaps it is in this implementation that TQM leads us on from practice planning (see Chapter 3) to the stage of developing the whole practice and its membership. Deploying skills without having developed the culture of team working will be ineffective, and the development of the practice culture and its structure is a key to quality improvement. But let us not forget that skills also are very important, and among them is audit — now in its rightful place as but one of several skills required to implement quality improvement, but nevertheless an important skill because it enables the evaluation of improvement in various chosen areas to be carried out.

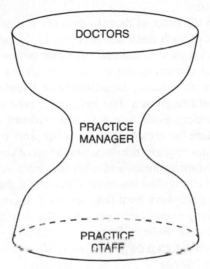

Fig. 9.5 Adapted with permission from the syllabus 'Improving health care quality'. Copyrighted by the National Development Project.

Implementation of quality improvement policies requires an enabling structure for the practice. Figure 9.4 offers such a framework, which can be contrasted with the management structure which is often found in general practice (Fig. 9.5) According to the traditional pattern doctors decide (with or without agreement); the practice manager rationalizes the decisions (sometimes having to pick out what appears to be best if the doctors' ideas conflict!) and implements them; and the staff do what they are told, with some feedback to or via the practice manager. With a good practice manager it *can* work, with a medium or poor practice manager it is a disaster: and with increasing demands and pressures being put on practices the failings of such management systems are increasingly apparent.

Contrast the structure in Fig. 9.4. The practice quality executive takes the lead in practice development. It may include all the partners or only some, but must be endorsed by all the partners. It will also contain representatives of some or all of the other key disciplines — practice nurse, practice manager, receptionist, and attached staff such as district nurse, health visitor, and midwife if appropriate. They will hear the views and opinions of all the members of the practice, using meetings and away-days and techniques such as brain storming or nominal group technique, to enable them to propose strategy. Having decided strategy, and the projects on which the practice intends to concentrate, they will appoint small teams with multidisciplinary representation (sometimes called quality improvement teams) to work on each project. The executive will brief the teams, set the timetable, and expect results and proposals from the teams, while taking the responsibility of ensuring the support and education that each team requires.

The teams take on the projects that the practice is working on. They should have a representative of each discipline involved in the process being reviewed, but may be very small. Just a doctor and dispenser might work on a formulary, or doctor, nurse, and clerical officer on cervical smears. Sometimes they will need to be larger, for instance if the handling of telephone systems were the problem. Teams should be given a clear brief and have extensive responsibility. They analyse the problem, collecting data and evidence as necessary; propose changes and procedure to remedy the problem; and crucially, evaluate the change. This evaluation requires the documentation of current practice, an idea of what would be an improvement, and after the implementation of change, re-measurement to see if change has occurred. Of course if the practice has an audit clerk then the team might work with that person, delegating a good deal of the data handling. In many ways this function in the quality improvement team corresponds to traditional audit, since they are indeed working on a topic, but with rather more emphasis on a deep analysis of the activity in order to identify the best direction for change.

The problem of jargon

Although this proposal for practice quality improvement is based on Total Quality Management (TQM) it is heavily adapted. In particular:

• 'Classical' TQM requires a great deal of measurement and statistical analysis, much more appropriate to industrial production than health care. In primary care we must never neglect measurement, but the statistics are less relevant.

• The 'teams' concept is rather over elaborate for primary care development. We have a limited amount of time and people, and a belief that many meetings of extensive teams are required is detrimental. Teams can be very small in primary care: but the teamwork principle is important.

• We have no 'bottom line'. In industry it is profits — or bust: with primary care it is a better service, often at increased cost. So we must be careful to readjust our concept of aims and rewards.

In addition the term 'TQM' tends to offend general practitioners. So perhaps 'Quality Improvement Methods for Primary Care': or 'Developing Practice Organization for Quality' are less threatening terms.

How does professional development take place?

A. Firstly quality improvement directs educational effort

Audit has tended to be carried out by a small number of people in a primary health care team, on an ad hoc basis. Many in the 'team' do not even know it is taking place. Using quality improvement methods, the practice has a strategy based on the needs of patients and the needs of the service. Everyone working in the practice should know this strategy, and their part in making it happen. This in its turn reveals areas where education is needed — whether it is members of the practice quality executive who need to learn about quality improvement methodology, or members of the quality improvement teams who need to learn about the topic on which they are working. No longer should the practice members merely attend the education that they enjoy, chosen from courses which others choose to put on — the educational need is driven by the requirement to provide a practice policy directed by patients' needs.

B. Secondly, all primary health care team members use their capabilities to the full

In the 'quality practice' all members of the organization have a role in determining strategy and understand the direction of development of the practice. All of them should constantly be considering how their own job can be done better. Many of them will be members of quality improvement teams. This helps the practice, because the plans and projects set up by the leaders now have a mechanism for implementation which involves those who have to work the resulting new protocols. It also helps the team members, because they can now feel that they are being heard, both their suggestions and their needs. It gives staff encouragement and opportunity to use their competencies, and indeed is an essential step in directing them and developing those competencies by education, both within the practice and on outside courses.

C. Quality improvement methods can be applied to the topic of professional development itself.

Both at practice and individual level the process of education should be regarded as an activity requiring a strategy and subject to review.

On a practice basis the leaders or the quality executive need to decide, in consultation with the primary health care team, a strategy for education — for example how important team education is and the areas in which it is required. Education may range from matters of access (Why is this important? What do others do? Where are the problems? Do we need communication training?), to clinical areas (What is the best management of patients with diabetes? What roles are required to provide good care?). The *culture* will then require agreement on protected time, costs, and payments, and recognition of achievement. The *techniques* required by the practice may range from tele-phone answering to stress reduction to asthma management.

On a personal level strategy is just as important. Once a person's role is established in the practice then their capacity to carry out that role needs to be assessed. This has a great deal of overlap with 'appraisal' and 'portfolio learning' (RCGP 1993). All team members, from the doctors to the clerks, need to assess in appraisal their competence to carry out their roles, and their educational needs to enable them to do better. Again strategy, culture (the time and energy spent) and techniques are good headings to consider.

D. Professionals and managers are able to work together

A quality improvement project has as its apex the practice's strategy, leading to a plan for the intermediate future. Health Authorities have an obligation to ensure high quality care for the populations for which they are responsible, and since they purchase primary care to achieve this they have an interest in such a plan, and indeed a right to be assured that the care they are purchasing is appropriate.

This gives great opportunity for co-operation between professionals and managers in agreeing appropriate care at strategic level. Health Authorities usually have greater public health awareness of population needs than primary care team members, while the primary care team is more aware of local need and feasibility of implementation. Agreeing strategic plans while leaving the practice flexibility for detailed implementation clearly gives huge scope for ensuring both good care and appropriate resources.

Since Authorities will wish to be assured of value for money an audit component to any plan will be essential. And high quality provision implies well trained staff, so assurance of an educational plan for the practice and its members is a logical requirement of any programme being purchased.

CASE STUDIES

1. A total quality management approach to diabetic care in general practice (Lawrence 1992)

In 1988 my practice decided to review the follow-up of patients with diabetes. We had done a good deal of audit but knew nothing of quality improvement theory. Table 9.1 shows our progress from 1988 to 1992 in achieving our aim of seeing each patient for a diabetes check a least once a year. (We also measured clinical processes and they improved as patients were regularly seen at their diabetic checks.)

Table 9.1 Performance of follow-up in diabetic patients

Year	No registered for follow-up	No. up to date with appointments		
		No recalled (%)	(% of recalled)	(% of registered)
1988	73	43(59)	18(42)	18(25)
1989	83	62(75)	31(50	31(37)
1991	76	66(87)	58(88)	58(76)
1992	82	82(100)	79(96)	79(96)

Of interest is the practice's processes in achieving this change. In 1988 the data were collected by one doctor and reported to a partners meeting and discussed. We did not set a plan. By 1989 improvement was marginal, and at this stage a team of doctor, nurse, and receptionist was set up, the process reviewed and plans made for improvement. This revealed:

Problem: A large part of the deficit was due to house-bound elderly.
   Plan: the district nurse would be involved in visiting regularly for diabetes checks.
Problem: Defaulting occurred due to difficulty with forward appointments
   Plan: One receptionist would take responsibility for this and send out reminder cards.

The receptionist, who had suggested the reminder system, also volunteered to collect the data for the following year and, (since in 1990 it sat on the doctor's desk for six months waiting to be analysed!), in 1991 she also offered to analyse and present it. It became one her main interests at work, and provided a great challenge to her to ensure that the practice offered a first class service. Clearly by 1991 things had greatly improved, but there were still deficiencies and it was agreed:

Problem: Half of the overdue patients were still house-bound.
   Plan: The practice nurse responsible for the diabetic clinic would go to these patients in their homes.
Problem: A few mobile patients still defaulted.
   Plan: Any patient found at audit to have defaulted would be notified to their usual doctor for follow-up.
By 1992 our follow-up success had reached 96%.

Professional development: As a result of this project professional development in the practice was considerable. The doctors were encouraged to look at clinical care, especially the relative merits of monitoring urinary glucose, fasting blood sugar, and HBA1C: they also reviewed their blood pressure management and retinoscopy. The nurses attended a course on lifestyle management for patients with diabetes and have developed their clinic management skills. And the receptionist developed audit skills (as a result of which she has left the practice, and is now the audit facilitator for the whole of Oxfordshire!).

2. Applying TQM to the education programme for internal medicine resident (Ellrodt 1993)

A decision was taken in July 1992 at Cedars Sinai Medical Centre in California to transfer significant programming responsibility for their education from the chief residents to the house officers. This was a decision taken by the senior members leading the Department of Medicine — the chief of medicine and the director of teaching. It was a conscious decision by the leadership to alter the culture of the department of medicine to involve house officers more in the design and development of their own teaching programme.

A Quality Improvement Committee was set up composed of elected leaders of the house staff, chief residents, and the director of the Internal Medicine teaching programme (Fig 9.6). This 'quality executive' was endorsed by and liaised with the chief residents (for education) and the Department of Internal Medicine (for clinical care). This contrasted with the previous system by which the house officers' education programme was organized by the chief resident who reported to the director of teaching who was responsible to the chief of medicine.

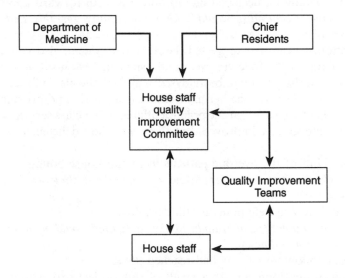

Fig. 9.6

A values statement to direct effort (Fig. 9.7) was developed by all the house staff at a retreat (while attending physicians looked after the hospital!) and unanimously endorsed. At subsequent workshops the house staff prioritized areas for improvement in the education programme. The topics were agreed by the Quality Improvement Committee which then set up and briefed teams to focus on such topics as ward teaching, electives, appropriate test organizing or ordering, orientation of new house staff and evaluation/feedback.

There was considerable concern in the department over giving such power to house staff, but in practice senior members have felt reassured. House staff have reorganized their work systems as well as looking at educational opportunity, and it is felt that education in the area of resource management is important, and only attainable in conjunction with responsibility.

Surveys of the house staff showed 68% felt that the rate of programme change was better, 63% that the training programme had improved, while only 3% felt that it had worsened after restructuring using TQM.

**Housestaff values Statement of
the Cedars-Sinai Medical Center
Internal Medicine Training Program**

We are committed to providing excellent and ever-improving care to our patients and our community:

To achieve this, we will:

- Foster mutual respect and support between all individuals at all levels

- Provide an educational environment that encourages ongoing life-long self-learning in collaboration with others

- Communicate 'evaluative information to others in a way that enables them to use it to their advantage'

- Expect responsibility and accountability in all interactions

- Embrace compassion, honesty, and trust between all individuals

- Nurture the individual for a leadership role in the community and the profession

- Appreciate the importance of the emotional, physical, and spiritual health of each individual

---

Fig. 9.7 Housestaff values statement.

3. Practice development using quality improvement methodology

A practice worked from two premises, one of which was a Health Centre shared with two other practices. The practice agreed to take part in a project run in Oxford Region in 1993/94 in which 19 practices agreed to apply TQM methods to practice development. Early in the development of the project the practice had an away-day, which began by eliciting practice members' concerns. They were:

- Lack of communication — split sites
- No feeling of team — uniprofessional working
- Low staff morale
- Lack of understanding of teamwork
- Lack of clearly defined objectives
- Lack of understanding each others' constraints
- Scepticism (we have tried it before)

Prior to the away-day a series of meetings had been held to identify priorities, 'this being the first attempt at priorities setting'. The topics perceived as needing most attention were:

- Nurses' appointment system
- Ordering of supplies
- In-house staff training
- Clarification of roles and responsibilities

It was decided to work on the nurses' appointment system, especially difficult because the nurses worked for all three practices. The Quality Improvement Team consisted of a practice manager from each practice, the leading practice nurse, and a doctor (who had been on a TQM introductory course). After monitoring the waiting times of patients and reviewing the work activity and length of time required for different procedures, changes were introduced including:

- Blocks of nurse time for specific activities
- Arrangements for 'fitting in' extras
- An attempt to book slots according to the time required
- Overlap working of nurses changing shifts

All this took place while the Health Centre was being rebuilt, and stress should have been heightened, but perceived advantages were:

- Planning and prioritizing on a multidisciplinary bases
- Communication within the team and between practices
- A feeling of involvement and better team working
- Less strain on the nurses working in the clinic

As a result the practice intends to move on a tackle a further problem using the same methodology, with receptionist, health visitor, district nurse, and doctor looking at the bereavement service.

A GUIDE FOR THOSE WHO WISH TO USE QUALITY IMPROVEMENT METHODS IN PRACTICE

A step-by-step guide to the introduction to Quality Improvement methodology is difficult! The breadth of the topic requires a book not a paragraph, and there is no good text on the subject for primary care. The essence has been expressed already in this chapter in the sections on 'the quality framework' and 'the quality practice', and the stages are as follows.

- The partnership must establish practice strategy and objectives
  — this probably requires an 'away-day' for the practice, and may need help from management consultants or FHSA facilitators
- The partners should appoint and endorse a practice quality executive
  — to oversee the development of quality in the practice and keep the programme up to time
- The quality executive should decide on priority topics for quality improvement, and establish and brief a multidisciplinary team to work on each chosen topic.
- Quality improvement teams work on their topics, evaluating the problem, involving patients, suggesting improvements, and reporting back to the executive.
- The partnership, through its executive, must endorse and implement the changes, communicating the issues and arranging training and education where required.

Most practices embarking on such a programme will require help. There are no readily accessible national courses in quality improvement methods for practices — perhaps because so much energy has been directed into audit. There are a few possibilities:

(a) The HEA runs team building workshops where practices are encouraged to send a small multidisciplinary group. The emphasis is on team building and communication, rather than the practical activity of quality improvement. For information try your local FHSA or write to the HEA Primary Care Unit, Churchill Hospital, Headington, Oxford.

(b) In the past courses in practice planning have been sponsored by Bristol Myers Squib and run by the BMS College.

 They emphasize strategic planning for partnerships, with less emphasis on implementation or team development . . . (none being run at the moment)

(c) For those who can afford it Donald Berwicks' course 'Improving Health Care Quality' run at Boston Massachusetts, is superb but expensive. Write to the Institute of Health Care Improvement, 1 Exeter Plaza, Boston, MA 021116, USA.

(d) Seminars are held around the country, and a Masters Course at the Department, by the University Department of Public Health Medicine at Hull. Write to Tricia Woollas, Director of Health Care Quality Programmes, Department of Public Health Medicine, University of Hull, HU6 7RX.

(e) A work book, QUALPAC, with facilitator support, has been developed by Karen Helme and John Marrin, with support from Gateshead FHSA. This course enables practices to work through the implementation of quality improvement with the benefit of local facilitation. In the process the practice develops strategies, a patients' charter, a business plan, staff development (almost 'Investors in People' standard), and service development. Either contact South of Tyne Health Commission, Horsely Hill Road, South

Shields: or the facility may be available through your local FHSA/Health Authority by the time this book is published.

(f) It is always worth contacting your local MAAG. They should know of local facilities for practice quality development.

REFERENCES

Bain, J. (1986). All good doctors should . . . *Journal of the Royal College of General Practitioners*, **36**, 249–51.

Berwick, D. M. (1989). Continuous improvement as an ideal in health care. *New England Journal of Medicine*, **320**, 53–56.

British Medical Association (1965). *Charter for the family doctor service*. BMA, London.

Crombie, D. L. and Fleming, D. M. (1988). Practice activity analysis. Occasional Paper 41 RCGP, London.

Deming, W. E. (1986). *Out of the crisis*. Massachusetts Institute of Technology, Cambridge MA.

Department of Health (1990). *Medical audit in the family practitioner services*. London. Department of Health, (HC(FP)(90)8).

Department of Health and Welsh Office (1989). General practice in the National Health Service. A new contract. HMSO, London.

Ellrodt, A. G. (1993). Introduction of TQM into an internal medicine residency. *Academic Medicine*, **68**, 817–23.

Humphrey, C. and Hughes, J. (1992). *Audit and development in primary care*. King's Fund Centre, London.

Lawrence, M. (1992). Audit and TQM in diabetic care in general practice. Quality in Health Care, 1992; 1 supplement: S 20–21 BMJ Publishing, London.

Lawrence, M. S. and Schofield, T. P. C. S. (eds) (1993). *Medical audit in primary health care*. Oxford University Press.

Lawrence, M. Griew, K., Derry, J., Anderson, J., and Humphreys, J. (1994). Auditing audit: Use and development of the Oxfordshire Medical Audit Advisory Group Rating System. *British Medical Journal*, **309**, 513–16.

Royal College of General Practitioners (1985a). *What sort of doctor?* Report from General Practice 23 RCGP, London.

Royal College of General Practitioners (1985b). Quality in General Practice. Policy statement 2. RCGP, London.

Royal College of General Practitioners (1993). Portfolio based learning in general practice. Occasional Paper 63. RCGP, London.

10 GP mentors — learning through counselling

David Whillier

What is the GP mentor? How does the mentor's role differ from that of the GP tutor, GP trainer, or others providing education for GPs? Where does counselling fit into professional education and development?

A summary of some of the literature concerning the modern mentor, its relationship to that of adult education and continuing professional education will be followed by the application of these ideas to Continuing Medical Education (CME) in general practice. An experimental GP mentoring project will be described before listing some of the lessons learnt.

INTRODUCTION

The mythology

In Homer's *Odyssey*, *Athene* the Greek goddess of wisdom guided Odysseus' son *Telemachus* in his search for his father who had not returned from the Trojan wars. Suitors, competing for the hand of his mother, *Penelope*, were disrupting the court. *Mentor* alone supported *Telemachus* who proposed a search for his father. *Athene* assumed the form of *Mentor*, an old and trusted friend of the family, to avoid overwhelming the young man. *Mentor*, representing this supernatural form of wisdom, did not accompany *Telemachus* on his journey, but always seemed to be there when needed. Although *Telemachus* did not bring his father back, he did discover that he was still alive and, with this very important discovery, proved himself, gaining status within the court.

The modern mentor

Daloz (1986), an American educationalist, explains the relevance of the mythology to the role of the modern mentor in education:

Mentors are guides. They lead us along the journey of our lives. We trust them because they have been there before. They embody our hopes, cast light on the way ahead, interpret arcane signs, warn us of lurking dangers, and point out unexpected delights along the way. There is a certain luminosity about them, and they often pose as magicians in tales of transformation, for *magic* is a word given to what we cannot see, and we rarely see across the gulf. As teachers we have much to learn from the mythology of the mentor.

He describes education as 'Transformational Journey'

. . . the task . . . is to reframe and understand in a radically new way the meaning of the world they once knew. This does not mean that the old world has been abandoned; rather it has been incorporated into a broader awareness of its place. It is *seen* in a new way. The journey does not take away our old experiences, as we often fear as we embark. It simply gives them new meaning.

. . . Our old life is still there, but its meaning has profoundly changed since we left home, seen from afar, and has been transformed by that vision. You can't go home again.

Adult education, the facilitator and the mentor

The concept of the 'Transformational Journey' incorporates, many of the now widely accepted principles of adult education. *Knowles* (1970) emphasizes the central role of the adult learner in respect of responsibility, motivation, the value of his experience, and continuous re-evaluation. *Perry* (1970) describes American college students' development from dualism or 'right answers' through uncertain relativism to commitment, again with recurring re-evaluation. *Rogers* (1969) proposes the innate ability of all humans to learn, provided the many barriers are removed, enabling 'Freedom to Learn'.

Brookfield (1986) lists *six principles of effective practice* in facilitating learning, which are paraphrased here, since they are widely accepted by those directly involved in adult education — often now described as *facilitators*.

1. Participation in learning is voluntary: adults withdraw if the learning does not *meet their needs* or make sense to them. Therefore what is to be learned should be appropriate and accessible.
2. Effective practice is characterised by a *respect* for the learner's self-worth. This does not rule out constructive criticism, but it does rule out practices that undermine confidence or belittle the learner.
3. Learning should be a *cooperative* venture between facilitator and learner, in collaboration. Leadership roles may be reversed at times.
4. Praxis is at the heart of effective facilitation. Praxis involves the engagement of learners and facilitators in a continual cyclical process of: activity → reflection upon activity → generating new activity and so on. ('Activity' does not exclude cognitive activity, e.g., exploring a completely new way of interpreting one's work.)
5. Facilitation aims to foster a spirit of *critical reflection* on professional, personal, and political life. Learners should understand that values, beliefs, and behaviours are culturally transmitted, provisional, and relative.
6. The aim of facilitation is the nurturing of *self-directed*, empowered adults; proactive, initiating individuals, in work, personal relationships, and in society.

These principles correlate well with Daloz's ideas of mentoring. What then are the differences between a facilitator and a mentor?

The processes involved are very similar and the distinction may be blurred, but it is the *context* which differs. Facilitators usually work with more than one learner and, of necessity, define a subject area in which they intend to work. Mentors *dedicate* a proportion of their efforts to individual learners and the initial direction of the process is determined by the latter. Facilitators often will be involved in the assessment of the students' progress, and these assessments may be used as surrogate measures of their effectiveness. Because the mentor is trying to guide by encouraging the removal of obstacles to learning, often private and personal, assessment or appraisal may seriously threaten the trust invested in the mentor. In this situation, assessment of effect of mentoring may become imprecise, unless the learner's occupation allows objective measurement of outcome, for example manufacturing output or sales.

The context of mentoring

The American psychologist Levinson *et al.* (1978) studied the lives of forty men; discovering that, during early adulthood, many had received support and guidance from older men who were usually less than a generation their senior. He reintroduced the term 'Mentor'.

Many have described the effect on performance of 'mentoring' particularly in business, education, and nursing. But few share a common definition of the modern mentor.

In her review of the literature, Jacobi (1991) identifies 15 diverse functions (see Table 10.1), reflecting three components of the mentoring relationship:

- emotional and psychological support
- direct assistance with career and professional development
- role modelling

Reviewing her list, the six functions highlighted seem to have particular relevance to continuing medical education (CME) in general practice. In most other cases, the mentor and mentee will share the same employer. The mentor will owe loyalty to both employer and mentee. The extent to which the mentor discharges his duties to his employer *indirectly*, that is by helping his mentee achieve his full potential, is likely to depend upon such factors as:

- the nature of the business or profession
- the structure and size of the organization
- the autonomy and seniority of the mentee

At one extreme, the 'mentor' to an entrant to a small hierarchical business may also have to *train* for specific tasks and further, to *assess* competence in these tasks. Her mentee may not feel inclined to trust his mentor if he perceives that judgements are being made that may affect his career prospects. At present, British GPs retain considerable autonomy and job security and are close to the other extreme. We should be aware that there may be difficulties in directly transposing mentoring models from other less autonomous professions such as nursing and teaching. In particular, the strengths of the mentoring relationship may be threatened if the mentor is seen to be involved in any assessments that may be used for re-accreditation.

Table 10.1 Jacobi's 15 mentoring functions

Acceptance/support/encouragement
Advice/guidance
Role model
Sponsorship/advocacy
Training/instruction
Information
Socialization/'host and guide'
Bypass bureaucracy/access to resources
Challenge/opportunity/'plum assignments'
Coaching
Protection
Visibility/exposure
Social status/reflected credit
Clarify value/clarify goals
Stimulate acquisition of knowledge

CONTRIBUTION TO PRACTICE

For many professions, undergraduate education involves the acquisition of its large specialized knowledge base, to a basic level. The mentor's role is gently to shift the focus of the practitioner's motivation to learn, from this unadulterated and rigorous science, to incorporate critically the contribution from personal experience.

The British GP gains professional autonomy with the acquisition of a registered list of patients. With this autonomy, comes responsibility for continuing education and development. Any 'career advancement' will be on the basis of *optional* extras to the GP's principal role, that is, the primary medical care of these patients. Because of the absence of any hierarchical structure within general practice, there is no senior or supervising doctor to plan and provide an individual practitioner's continuing education during a career that may span another 45 years. If, as Schön (1987) suggests, professionals *personally* modify research-based knowledge for application in the 'swampy ground' of practice, such a directive educational supervisor would be inappropriate. The idea of mentorship is appealing in this situation.

However, much of the stimulus to all educational activity before achievement of professional autonomy as a GP can be considered as primarily external. High achievement at school is followed by the potentially stressful acquisition of a large knowledge mass in preparation for the final qualifying examinations. Even before Vocational Training became compulsory in 1981, it was accompanied by financial inducement in the form of the Vocational Training Allowance. One of the effects of summative or end-point assessment will be to reinforce external motivation to learn. A young doctor taking his first steps as an independent practitioner may well cling to the familiar educational culture, that is, being *told* by expert specialists.

Many entrants to general practice during the last 25 years will have experienced aspects of a mentoring relationship with trainers who have attempted to engender trust, to encourage lifelong learner-centred, self-directed learning, and to offer professional and personal support. But, the experience of this type of relationship is not universal and many, who entered general practice before 1977, had no formal general practice based education. This is not to suggest that these GPs, as a group, are not well developed practitioners who take their responsibility for self-directed learning very seriously, rather that *some* may have difficulties, having been *conditioned* by the specialist undergraduate teachers to consider 'keeping up to date' as beyond their grasp. Furthermore, some experienced GPs will find the idea of mentoring more familiar than others. Even those who have regarded their trainers as mentors need to make adjustments. A hierarchical gap, however small will have existed — the trainee has been 'allowed' to treat the patients of a senior doctor, who has retained overall responsibility, and has to certify the trainee's educational achievement as satisfactory.

Against this background, several qualities of the relationship between GP and mentor emerge.
1. Trust
   In their relationship, an autonomous GP must trust his* mentor to have only his interests at heart. He must believe that their discussions are confidential, that is, they will not provide gossip and will not be used to put the GP's livelihood at risk, for example in re-accreditation.
2. Empathy
   The GP and mentor must have a shared understanding of the job. GPs may believe that only another GP will have sufficient understanding to act as his mentor.
3. Learner centredness
   The mentor will need the humility to believe that others have experiences and insights into the job just as valid as her* own and that their learning and development will occur by reflection on these experiences and insights and subsequent experimentation.
4. Wisdom
   The GP must perceive the mentor as bringing sufficient 'wisdom' to the relationship to make it fruitful, but without hierarchical distance. *Athene*

---

* For brevity alone, the female gender of the force behind the original *Mentor (Athene)* is used and the traditional male gender of the GP.

assumed the form of the original *Mentor* to the same end. The mentor will often require seniority and reputation, but the ability to understand and make sense of the GP's ideas may be seen as an indication of wisdom.

The 'Transformational Journey' of a GP's professional lifetime of 30 or 40 years may be considered to involve at least three interdependent areas of change.

1. Development of scientific knowledge — 'recent advances'
   Important though many medical discoveries have been to general practice, the traditional 'family doctor' role of the first part of the century seems to be valued (and sometimes missed) by many patients
2. Changes of the place of the profession in a developing society
   The profession of medicine developed from apothecaries and barber surgeons, gaining its status in the eighteenth century. Patient awareness and more recently consumerism may be seen as threatening this, although the status of British general practice within the medical profession has increased considerably during the last 40 years.
3. Movement through the stages of a personal life
   The personal changes experienced during a professional lifetime — marriage, parenthood, loss of parents, and preparation for retirement — are surely more intense than changes in medical knowledge or society.

Cartwright (1967) reports GPs' expressions of tedium of their work suggesting a paucity of external change. Maybe GP mentors should see themselves as helping to guide *personally changing* practitioners through relatively static professional demands.

. . .Our old life is still there, but its meaning has profoundly changed since we left home, seen from afar, and has been transformed by that vision.

(Daloz)

AN EXAMPLE OF GP MENTORING:
THE SOUTH EAST THAMES PROJECT

In 1989, ten GPs were appointed as mentors to be linked to half of the twenty postgraduate centres in the South East Thames Health Region, an area which encompasses the counties of Kent, East Sussex, and the South East quadrant of London. This would be an experimental group of GPs who would assist both the organizers and providers of CME within the region, and those to whom it was aimed — established GPs. Each mentor would relate to the GP tutor and others involved with CME in the Health District: Clinical Tutor, RCGP Tutor, in and outside the Postgraduate Centre. He or she would have the task of offering to visit *each* of the one hundred or so GPs in the district, to spend about one hour facilitating the GP's own identification of learning needs, and to provide him with a written summary of their meeting. The mentor's prime task would *NOT* be to provide detailed information to the providers of courses, neither would he act as a 'postman' between GPs and the GP tutor. Rather, he or she would be *empowering* local GPs to identify their educational needs and communicate them to these providers. However insights of the process of learning by local GPs might well be a valuable contribution to the District Postgraduate planning committees and others organizing CME.

Appointment of the mentors

The mentors were chosen on the basis of enthusiasm for the concept of mentoring and qualities of personal sensitivity rather than educational experience. All of the eleven GPs who applied for the ten posts were male, although we had hoped that women would apply. The organizers of a future project should consider how they might encourage female GPs to apply.

Mentor training and support

The mentors first met and formed a cohesive group at a two day residential induction. The educational adviser provided basic interview skill training. They were introduced to the duality of the mentor's role in this project.
• provision of a *service* to a group of GPs
• *research* into the feasibility of providing this innovative and exploratory, but ill-defined service

Three recurring themes appeared during this first weekend, and continued to surface, although with decreasing intensity, throughout the project:
• a tension between mentors *imposing* themselves on GPs and the possibility that they might be *unprepared* to deal with problems uncovered, particularly those of a serious and personal nature
• the degree of *structure* appropriate to the various stages of the mentoring process and, allied to this, the *breadth* of the definition of 'education' in this context
• *confidentiality* of their reports, and their use for research

Table 10.2 The six stages of GP mentoring in this project

---

1. Arranging the interview
2. Preparation or 'homework' by the GP
3. The interview
4. Writing the report
5. The report and feedback questionnaire sent to GP for comments
6. Amended report, GP questionnaire and mentor feedback sent to project coordinator

---

The mentor group produced initial guidelines and instruments to be used in the six stages of the mentoring process listed in Table 10.2. It should be noted that these stages might be considered preliminary to a longer-term and more involved mentoring relationship.

The GP's 'homework' was an attempt to stimulate thoughts about personal learning by keeping a simple '*Learning diary*' which included the following:

During the week before we meet please write down up to six new or ongoing problems you face in your life as a GP and any methods you may have used to cope with them.

Did you undertake any other learning activities during this week? Please list and comment freely below.

Was this an unusual week for you? If so how?

They agreed on these topic headings for the semi-structured report of the mentor's meeting with the GP — '*My notes on our meeting*'.

(The learning diary)

1. Past experience of medical education
2. What learning means to you
3. How you maintain enthusiasm
4. How you find time — priorities

'*GP's comments*' were to be requested when the report was sent to the GP for possible amendment.

In order to assist my development as a mentor I should value some feedback on our recent meeting and my notes on it.

1. What did you think of the interview and these notes?
2. What came out of the interview for you?
3. What further thoughts have you had about education and learning since we met?

The *Mentor's comments* on the interview were recorded in two stages:

My immediate reaction to the meeting

My reaction to the GP's comments

At a second residential meeting, two years later, the mentors devised guidelines for the appointment and induction of their successors with enthusiasm.

They suggested the following qualities:

● experience
● local knowledge
● reputation
● adaptable but non-judgemental listening style
● ability to summarize and organize
● ability to learn in a group
● enthusiasm, optimism, and resilience

After the proposed 'mentoring' by an experienced mentor, they suggested that induction should be continued at a residential meeting which included:

- Discussion of the mentor's role — 'reality vs expectation'
- Practical small group tasks — setting up interview, letters, etc.
- Video presentation of a mentor interview, demonstrating styles, skills, pitfalls
- Role play and video feedback, with leaders as 'standard' interviewees
- Confirming commitment by 'signing on' in light of new insights into the mentor's role

Throughout the interviewing stage of the project, the mentors and the project leaders held half day meetings at approximately 3–4 monthly intervals. These meetings had three broad aims:

- to maintain the cohesion and mutual support of the mentors' group
- to discuss their progress and their current understanding of the mentoring role
- to share and develop solutions to problems, practical and others,

Several mentors reported feelings of *isolation* between meetings. The group arranged to combat this by forming two local groups to meet more frequently. One expressed 'running out of steam [when the group met less frequently]' another found it 'difficult to restart'. A third found that his struggling had eased 'when x [another mentor] wrote me a letter'. A regular newsletter was suggested by two of them.

At least initially, most mentors expressed the need for more feedback, at least initially, both from the centre and in particular from the GPs they had visited. Although at least three stated in their final interviews that the former was no longer required and that it was unrealistic to expect this additional burden on the GP.

CASE STUDIES

None of the mentors in the S.E. Thames project completed all the interviews required by the original research design — two mentors withdrew from the project. one very early on, the other, later, because of family illness. The overall completion rate of 23% included a very wide variation of achievement, which was associated with the 'reputation' of the mentor, that is his *seniority, status* (in relation to involvement in CME or medical politics), and the *location* of his practice in the same district. Three of the GPs visited made the following comments.

'I didn't believe a mentor who did not know me would have gained so much inside knowledge'

'The interview [was] relaxed and enjoyable. Conducted by a friend of long standing gave an advantage — an understanding of the ethos behind one's life's work against which the outcome could be set. The disadvantage must have been a reluctance to be critical, challenging or rude.'

'It is rare to have the opportunity for an hour to think about and discuss **my** [CME] and related wider issues. Being facilitated by someone with your experience and ability enhanced its value . . .'

Two of the most negative comments came from older GPs who alluded to the inexperience of their young mentors. However the high completion rate of one of the young mentors may have been related to his clear agenda and strong views on CME.

Arranging the interview

One mentor's secretary arranged most of his interviews, without apparent difficulty. The remainder contacted the GP personally, sharing practical advice and gaining confidence in the support meetings. They found most GPs unaware of the project or of the mentor's role in the early months. The mentors themselves had yet to attain a clear definition, but they would have welcomed more intensive advertising at this stage. The GPs who agreed to the interview were representative of the GP population of the region in terms of age, gender, ethnicity, and practice size. Aware of the research element of the project, most mentors initially approached GPs on a random basis. They soon agreed that, while gaining confidence with their task, GP acquaintances would provide a less stressful clientele. However all mentors had interviewed GPs previously unknown to them, by the end of the project.

The mentoring interview

The mentors usually conducted interviews on the GP's 'own ground', in the surgery or at home, at a mutually convenient time during the working day or later. Some suggested that advantages, such as conviviality and freedom from interruption, might be countered by the danger that the exchanges would be more superficial, social rather than professional. Ideally, the mentor should explicitly encourage the GP to make this choice of location.

The mentors intended the one hour interview to be informal, relaxed, and non-threatening. Most soon lost their reservations concerning 'imposition' on the GPs they visited and realized that, on the whole, GPs usually welcome the unusual opportunity to talk to a colleague whose agenda is focused on themselves. For example

'I appreciated talking to an independent GP, more like an observer, who from his experience could understand what I feel'

The structure and control exerted by the mentor in the interview obviously influenced its content. Many doctors were keen to talk about how they viewed their practices (especially the considerable administrative changes relating to the new contract), their partners, their patients, and the everyday stresses of the job and its interaction with life outside medicine. The mentors continued to question the relevance of such mundane issues to *education*, although with decreasing frequency. The breadth of the term and the 'legitimacy' of including personal 'baggage' was central to their definition of the mentor's role. The mentor clearly needed a clear understanding of the *boundary* between his role and that of counsellor or therapist.

The mentor's report

Within a week of the interview, each mentor sent the GP a type-written report of around 600–700 words on two sides of A4 paper. The mentors took report writing very seriously, spending between one and a half and two hours to describe the one hour interview.

No mentor was unaffected when a doctor questioned or amended aspects of his report or responded negatively. One or two reacted strongly, either by tightening up the conduct of interviews or spending even longer writing the reports. However, more often, the mentors were congratulated on the comprehensiveness and accuracy of their reports.

I'm amazed by the notes — you seem to know me better than I know myself . . . you distilled the essence of what I was trying to say . . .

GPs' views about the value of mentoring

Nearly all (90%) of the GPs interviewed gave written feedback after receiving their mentors' reports. A selection of their comments follows.

(i) Present situation and future CME

Showed me just how fed up I am with things at present and how negative I am being. Perhaps the GP mentor arrangement should evolve as a regular counselling service to GPs who wish to avail themselves of help and advice from fellow GPs who can indicate obvious problems not apparent to the individual.
By verbalizing one's personal thoughts on education, etc. (with the help of a mentor) it seemed to move the process on a step or two towards action.

(ii) Past education and present needs

Needed to be persuaded to begin with. Helped me examine my own ideals again and to attempt some kind of assessment as to how I match up to them in reality.
I was most excited about the way it made me look at and consider my professional development in a way that I never had done before.
Searching interview coupled with a historical review.

(iii) Role and effect of mentor

Mentor a good catalyst. Ventilated a few well sublimated feelings.

Found myself summarizing my whole professional life and attitudes — I don't think I've done that before.

The mentor should help set goals with time limits to enable jobs to get done (always meaning to do them).

The strange thing I noticed was that . . . there was a sort of therapeutic element. I felt better after the interview than I had done before. Why this happened I do not know.

(iv) Importance of CME

I am now aware that there may be a place for more organized PG study, locally. Should support local PG centre more.

Need to do research with a colleague group.

Realized I should do a programme of studies (e.g. MA at Guy's).

Showed me . . . you can continue to learn from day to day experiences if you have time to sit back and digest them, and possibly also if you discuss them with a peer.

From the 185 doctors who expressed a view on the value of the mentoring process,

- 80% valued it very or fairly highly
- 15% did not value it very highly
- 5% did not attach any value at all to the experience

The main reasons given, by the 80%, *for finding the experience valuable* were classified by Ellie Chambers, an independent researcher, as follows. Some doctors gave more than one reason.

(i) *Stocktakers* Over a third of these doctors agreed with one who said that mentoring provided '*a chance to take stock of the present situation, and future prospects*' with regard to CME.

(ii) *Reflectors* Almost a third of them said it was '*interesting*' or '*stimulating*' to have the opportunity to think about one's own past education and present needs.

(iii) *Confiders* A quarter of the doctors said that it was good to talk to someone outside one's own practice, someone sympathetic who was also knowledgeable about General Practice: for a small group of them it was '*therapeutic*', and more a matter of having a mentor to '*turn to*' or '*moan to*', and to help them identify problems and seek possible solutions to them.

(iv) *Responders* A fifth of them responded well to the experience because it reminded them about the importance of CME, making them want to become more involved. They recognized the need to keep up to date, through reading or attending meetings at the Post Graduate Centre; also, a number of them supported the view that '*it helped me to think about what I can learn in day-to-day surgeries*'.

Reasons given for the lukewarm response of the 15% included the failure of the mentor to provide guidance or *'answers'* and conversely, disagreement with the mentor's views on CME. Some doctors clearly judged the process a luxury in their extremely crowded schedules. Of the 5% who were dismissive of or hostile to mentoring, two older doctors commented on their mentor's age and lack of experience. One doctor reacted very defensively to his interview report which he perceived as critical.

The mentor's role

As already mentioned, the mentors sought a clearer understanding of their role throughout the project. Their interview reports, along with the feedback forms provided evidence of the various functions that mentors performed, and their preferred styles of mentoring. The five mentoring functions extracted from Jacobi's list (p. 116) form the basis of the analysis in Table 10.3.

Table 10.3 Identification of mentor functions

Function	No. of mentors
1. Providing acceptance, support, encouragement	7
2. Offering advice or guidance	6
3. Providing information	3
4. Helping to clarify values/goals	7
5. Stimulating the acquisition of knowledge	5

The *styles* exhibited by the mentors varied in relation to these functions. At one end of the spectrum lay non-judgemental summarizing and *reflection* of the GP's concerns back for further consideration, at the other, strong *recommendations* related to the mentor's personal view of CME. Half of the mentors' styles tell between these extremes of directiveness, with the mentors providing advice, guidance, or information where they considered it appropriate.

The mentor's summary of the GP's experience of education and learning, past and present and included differing degrees of interpretation.

You would have liked to have been encouraged to attend more clinics in the minor specialities and had hands on experience to boost your confidence and expertise.
You always wanted to be a GP in rural practice . . . 'hands on' ward clerking, with student responsibility for patient care. This sort of teaching suited you well.
You learn from consultants by direct contact, and through their letters, when they are informative! I have the impression that these sources are not as good as they have been
. . . You have always been dysnumerate, and for this reason felt ill at ease with Diabetes when the counting of Insulin units seemed a hurdle.

I suspect that your admission of clinical insecurity is a part of your personality rather than a reflection on your education — it keeps you on your toes and stops you becoming complacent or dismissive of problems. It also allows you to attend courses looking at common problems which make up the vast percentage of our work.

Some mentors provided a neutral summary of the GP's future educational plans, others offered interpretation. Some went further and made broad, or even specific, suggestions.

As for the future, you had no fantasies but were happy now to look for challenges. Your educational experiences of the later years had made you much happier now to both confront and deal with challenges than you would have been with such 'problems' in your younger years.
When the time comes that you feel more settled, it looks as if becoming a trainer will provide you with both interest and a new challenge. If at some stage you are able to have a sabbatical, you would find that an interesting experience and probably would attempt to take it in the third world, time allowing.
You have an ambition to become a trainer . . . You always feel the need to have a goal but would be wise not to over extend yourself . . .
I suspect from the way the interview went, that you are sometimes quite isolated in your practice . . . Are there other ways in which you could find support outside the practice?
You seem to be suffering badly from too much to do and not enough time to talk or to think . . . it seems perverse to suggest that you need to give up more free time to sort things out, but I would suggest to you that in the short term this may actually be necessary.

The process of preparing reports for the GPs they had interviewed was central to the project. As well as providing a summary of expressed needs for the GP's benefit, it allowed the mentor to reflect on the developing definition of his role, his understanding of medical education and, sometimes, his perception of himself as a general practitioner. For example, one said:

'I was very interested in the pattern and depth of experience of this doctor, and the way in which this experience had been built up'

another simply that

'his [the doctor's] comments have helped me'.

A third remarked, somewhat wryly,

'I am glad that she thought the interview was worthwhile and also that she wishes to organize her time more productively. It is something which I should do as well'.

One said,

'Yet again the "mentoring" process facilitated sharing of some very personal problems and hang ups. It is proving to be a humbling experience'.

another demonstrated his application of psychological theory,

'These interviews confirm my admiration for construct theory — each interviewee makes sense of General Practice in his own way'.

another, his understanding of local GP education,

'Clarified many points for me regarding local GPs' dissatisfaction with local PG meetings etc'.

There seemed to be a development or 'maturation' of the mentors during the three years. This seemed to be similar to the process, described by Perry and quoted above in relation to the application of mentoring CME. The mentors themselves were becoming '*professionalized*'. One of the older members of the group said that he was

'more confident to be paddling in a large pool, unsure of the geography'

Outcomes for PGEA organizers — the content of the reports

Attitudes to previous medical education
Less than one-fifth of the 86% of GPs who discussed it said they had so enjoyed the earlier, academic aspects of their education that they missed hospital doctoring.

Attitudes to general practice
80% of the GP's interviewed expressed feelings of stress related to increased workload, for 16% this was a major intrusion into their personal lives. Many were disillusioned by the changes in GP ethos brought about by the (new) 1990 GP contract, in particular the emphasis on administration and finance, 7% were so thoroughly disenchanted that they were planning to leave general practice. Another 30% had mixed feelings. The reasons for the negative attitudes of these two groups are summarized in table 10.4.

Table 10.4 Reasons for negative attitudes to general practice

Feeling of 'Burn-out'	25%
Practice management including fundholding and computerization	18%
Problems with partners	13%
Feelings of isolation	8%

Of the 63% with a more positive attitude to practice, two thirds agreed that practice management and computer training was needed. One third mentioned appreciation, sometimes grudging, of the stimulation of the New Contract

Attitudes to CME

Not surprisingly, the new Postgraduate Educational Allowance was mentioned by many GPs. Some resented the financial motivation of the new system. But others commented that, while educational time had been eroded by clinical and other work, the new allowance might protect educational time within the practice. Only 20% considered their current practice arrangements adequate. Almost all the GPs revealed *preferred learning methods*.

41% said that their learning was mainly based on *experience*: much of their current learning was *opportunistic* and based on analysis of *patients' problems*, with follow-up reading and research done in order to find solutions.

'Learning is to do with increasing knowledge through experience'.

23% said that their learning was mainly *compensatory*: they took steps to acquire what they needed to fill *gaps* in their knowledge, and concentrate their efforts on strengthening areas of weakness.

20% said they regarded learning as a *life-long* process, which goes on all the time in a wide *variety* of ways.

41% of all these doctors thought that their education and training should be *more GP-focused*.

Many GPs questioned the value of small group work and discussion, mainly because of lack of structure and clear objectives. **30%** said they particularly valued *specialized lectures*. The mentor group discussed this view which countered their view of adult education. One blamed the GPs' familiarity with this type of education.

'the teaching of adults was still in its infancy, and the vast majority of teaching was done as didactic lectures'

These GPs' comments underline the theme of this book: a move from teacher-based education of doctors to a learner-centred and broadly based approach. Two types of *motivation for CME* were recorded:

- to improve their knowledge and skills in order to offer patients better quality of care and better, more efficient, service;
- to keep up-to-date with advances in medicine/keep abreast of their colleagues in hospital medicine, for their own satisfaction and for the ultimate good of patients.

Their current CME involvement is shown in Table 10.5: most doctors were involved in more than one activity.

Many GPs noted the value of contact with colleagues but, perhaps not surprisingly, there was no clear preference for the timing and duration of postgraduate centre meetings.

Only one third had no definite plans for their future CME. 15% had already acted on plans between the mentor interview and receipt of the report.

Table 10.5 Doctors' current involvement in CME

Activity	% involved
Reading medical journals	84%
Attending local meetings/courses with colleagues (eg Young Principals groups, 'clubs', 'societies')	63%
Attending meetings at the local PG Centre	53%
GP Trainer (local PGC and/or trainee-practice)	45%
Attending clinical practice meetings with partners	37%
Attending residential/short courses outside region	35%
Attending drug company presentations or sponsored meetings	12%

STEP-BY-STEP GUIDE

1. Preparation

(a) Aims

The organizers will need to agree the general ethos of the service, although the mentors should gradually develop personal and group understanding of their role within this ethos. As discussed in the first section, mentors in other professions have been involved in appraisal. However, in the project described, the aim was to help the GP to reflect on the content and style of his learning needs and to help him discover barriers to meeting them. The mentors attempted this by summarizing one hour lightly structured interviews with individual GPs. Because the barriers to learning might be of a confidential or personal nature, the process required that the mentor should be trusted by the GP. If a similar project were to offer repeated interviews, the ethos would also include the mentor's trust that the GP would wish to meet these educational needs (or developments of them) without the need for their formal review.

(b) Funding

This is considered in detail later.

(c) Liaison

The organizers should take care to liaise with other GP professional bodies that may consider aspects of the mentor's role to be their own. To aid planning, GP tutors may be assessing the GPs' learning needs in similar or different ways. Broad definition of learning and education by mentor may impinge on the pastoral support offered to local GPs by the Local Medical Committee, local British Medical Association division, or the faculty of the Royal College of

General Practitioners. Certainly a mentor with this view will need to be aware of such local resources.

(d) Publicity

If the mentors are to be selected as peers of the GPs who will be offered the service, the latter should be aware of the aims of the service before applications for the posts are sought. Rumour, speculation, and misinformation are almost inevitable as the project starts, but attempts to minimize the perceived threat to GPs may be assisted by the liaisons mentioned above.

2. Appointment

The organizers will need to decide on the degree of peer GP involvement in the mentoring service. A shared understanding of the GP's job may encourage trust, but others, such as educationalists or psychologists may have better counselling skills and educational knowledge. It is likely that both groups will be represented in the organizing group. The organizers should explore ways of encouraging female applicants to apply, perhaps by talking with female GP groups.

The list of desirable mentor qualities agreed by the South East Thames group is comprehensive.

- experience
- local knowledge
- reputation
- adaptable but non-judgemental listening style
- ability to summarize and organize
- enthusiasm, optimism, and resilience

They would have welcomed an interview by an experienced mentor before 'signing on'.

3. Training and support

At the start of the project, the agendas of the new mentors and the organizers are likely to require a one to two day meeting. They may include:

- Formation of the group
- Introduction to interviewing/counselling skills
- Exploration of the mentor's role
- Confidentiality and responsibility
- Practical issues, e.g. agreement of forms, how to approach GPs

The mentors described were encouraged to develop a group understanding of their role. They discussed this repeatedly at quarterly half-day support meetings, particularly in terms of the breadth of the definition of education — their boundaries — and how much advice they should offer. At these meetings they also shared problems of access to GPs, conducting the interview and report writing. They expressed feelings of isolation and lack of motivation between the meetings and probably this interval should not be exceeded. A newsletter and local sub-groups, particularly if several mentors are appointed to a district, might reduce the potential for isolation. Eventually, an experienced group of mentors is likely to gain the confidence to develop and treasure individual styles.

Report writing is both time consuming and foreign to most GPs. However, it was central to the project described. The GPs interviewed commented on the value and accuracy of most reports, but the reports also served to heighten the mentors' understanding of general practice, professional education, and the mentoring process. Feedback from both GPs and mentors was used as research data, but it too seemed to assist mentor development.

4. Access to GPs

Careful continued publicity and liaison should lessen the threat of an approach by a GP mentor. News of the successful (and unsuccessful) interviews will be spread by word of mouth. However, the inducement of Postgraduate Education Allowance credits may encourage some GPs to 'take the plunge'.

5. Funding

The South East Thames mentors used at least three hours for arranging, travelling, undertaking, and writing up a one hour GP interview. Some achieved three interviews during two half day sessions. Five half days each year for training and support seems a bare minimum. A mentor probably needs a minimum concentration of experience of one interview each month to allow training and development Although a single mentoring experience has been shown to be acceptable to GPs, most mentors and many GPs expressed the wish for a second visit within a year or two. Several GPs said they would have preferred a choice of mentors. These estimates allow predictions of workload. For example, one hundred GPs offered a meeting with one of a choice of three mentors every year would probably involve 81 (2/3 × 100 + 5 × 3 training) half day sessions per year divided between the three mentors, or a minimum of 27 each. It is of course possible that the annual visit would represent an average, that some GPs would wish more frequent contact, some less.

As previously stated, the mentors gained insights into general practice and professional education. These insights might be considered valuable preparation for future organizers of CME. Such insights could also be used by trainers in preparing their trainees both for life-long learning as GP principals and for the variety of general practice outside their own training practices. 'Fallow' GP Trainers may be considered as a group of potential mentors. Perhaps an FHSA might consider funding a pilot scheme on this basis.

6. Evaluation

Outcome measures for general practice are notoriously difficult. Those aspects that are easily evaluated objectively, often involving preventative measures, referrals to hospital, and prescribing are not necessarily those of most importance to the patients; those in *Schön's* 'swampy lowland of practice'. Clearly the difficulties extend to evaluating the effect of a mentoring service on these outcomes. The attempts at overcoming these difficulties for possible *re-accreditation and re-certification* may allow investigation of effects of a mentoring service, but as stated above, mentors risk destroying their GPs' trust and confidence, if they are seen to be participating in this type of assessment. The prime function of accreditation or re-accreditation seems to be the protection of an unsuspecting public from GPs they are unable to identify as so seriously deficient that they should lose their professional autonomy. Professional development is based upon this autonomy. Mentors will help those who feel threatened by the assessments, and those failing them, but they should never be seen as 'policing' them.

Portfolio-based learning

Clearly the qualities and roles of the mentor in portfolio-based learning are similar to those described in Chapter 8. However there are subtle but significant differences. A successful portfolio-based learning cycle involves the demonstration that agreed, defined, and planned educational objectives have been achieved. To maintain learner autonomy, self-assessment is the method of choice. The mentor encourages and facilitates the identification and achievement of the objectives. It is the *clarity* of the objectives that may distinguish the two types of mentoring. This clarity is helpful to those outside the process — the paymasters of GP and mentor, for example. But the 'Transformational Journey' is broken into small attainable steps, of necessity defined in terms meaningful before the steps are taken. The whole 'journey' often includes changes of a depth that involve a development of the way in which knowledge, medicine, and the GP's role are perceived. Obviously these changes are not excluded by portfolio-based learning, but there is a danger that during the defined learning activity this depth of change can threaten the objectivity of the portfolio and vice versa.

However, evaluation difficulties should not deter enthusiasm for the concept of mentoring which is soundly based on accepted principles of adult and continuing education. They have not deterred the continued enthusiasm of many GPs for their work which is no less resistant to evaluation.

REFERENCES

Brookfield, S. D. (1986). *Understanding and facilitating adult learning*. Open University Press, Buckingham.

Cartwright, A. (1967). *Patients and their doctors: a study of general practice.* Routledge and Kegan Paul, London.

Daloz, L. A. (1986). *Effective teaching and mentoring: realizing the transformational power of adult learning experiences.* Jossey-Bass, San Francisco.

Jacobi, M. (1991). Mentoring and undergraduate academic success: a literature review. *Review of Educational Research,* **61**, 4, 505–32.

Knowles, M. S. (1970). *The modern practice of education: from pedagogy to andragogy.* Cambridge Book Company.

Levinson, D. J., Carrow, C. N., Klein, E. B., Levinson, M. H., and McKee, B. (1978). *The seasons of a man's life.* Ballantine Books, New York.

Perry, W. G. (1970). *Forms of intellectual and ethical development in the college years.* Holt, Reinhart and Winston, New York.

Rogers, C. (1969). *Freedom to learn.* Charles E. Merrill, Columbus.

Schön, D. A. (1987). *Educating the reflective practitioner.* (Second edition). Jossey-Bass, San Francisco.

11 Specialty Liaison Groups

Andrew Willis

INTRODUCTION

The purpose of Specialty Liaison Groups (SLGs) is to encourage two-way communication between GPs and specialists in order to make the best use of available resources. They seek to do this in two ways.

(i) By informing GPs of the services available within secondary care and the manner in which these can be most effectively used. The production of locally agreed clinical guidelines is an important element of this exercise.

(ii) By informing specialists of areas of local hospital and community services that produce particular difficulty for GPs or their patients. This utilizes the role of all GPs as direct or indirect purchases of secondary services.

Whilst the primary purpose is to affect service provision across the primary/secondary care interface. SLGs have the potential to improve the provision of primary care by influencing the way in which GPs make referrals.

This chapter begins by discussing the ideas behind SLGs and the changing climate within the NHS that makes them particularly relevant now. It then considers their contribution to health care, both in theoretical terms and by describing three examples of their use. Following this the chapter provides a step-by-step guide to implementing SLGs before closing with a discussion of how the concept may be extended to form the very core of District and locality commissioning.

THE IDEAS BEHIND SLGS

SLGs are a simple approach to helping specialists and GPs work together to provide high quality, effective clinical services that are sensitive to the needs of local communities. *En passant* they encourage clinicians to recognize the costs, benefits, and opportunity-costs of their actions. It is this last concept that is often overlooked by doctors trained, mistakenly, to believe that 'clinical freedom' is synonymous with freedom from cost consideration. In reality the decision to do one thing may preclude the doing of something else and it is the appreciation of opportunity-costs that offers most scope for service development across the purchaser–provider interface.

Managing demands that exceed the available resources is a problem that has to be addressed by clinicians within any system of health care. The task might be eased by the addition of more resources but it would not be eliminated. SLGs present a forum within this background for clinicians to bring their influence to bear on health service planning. They do not avoid the political debate concerning resources for the NHS; they simply bypass it as being something beyond the primary remit of clinicians. It is for politicians and civil servants to determine resource allocations and to be accountable to the public for any consequential rationing. It is for clinicians and local managers to use the resources available to them as effectively as possible. SLGs help them do so.

This chapter recognises the NHS District and any constituent Localities as the basic unit of population for health service planning. As Regional Health Authorities disappear and the FHSAs and DHAs coalesce into joint commissioning authorities it is to District populations that resources will be distributed for the purposes of planning and accountability. There are commonly long-standing working relationships between specialists and GPs within the catchment areas of local hospitals. A simple approach for bringing benefits to overall patient care is to enhance these traditional links through SLGs.

WHAT ARE SLGS?

SLGs were conceived in Northampton during 1990 as small groups of two or three GPs and a similar number of specialists working together concerning a particular clinical discipline. The groups promote two-way communication. On the one hand an obvious outcome is the production of clinical guidelines for GPs to be incorporated in postgraduate education programmes. On the other, GPs can discuss with specialists the ways in which they would like hospital and community services developed (Fig. 11.1). This is merely good professional practice, regardless of the level of funding obtained. It does not reduce the need for identifying short falls in services and lobbying for the resources to meet them. On the contrary, it assists that activity.

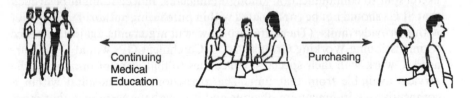

Continuing Medical Education Purchasing

Fig. 11.1

Experience shows that the role of GPs as direct or indirect purchasers can be left to underpin such discussions. An overt 'purchaser' focus from GPs is usually unnecessary and may cause friction between clinical colleagues who rely upon each other within their day to day work. It would be no triumph to remove the despotic specialists of the past only to replace them with anarchic GPs who load public money into their egocentricaly aimed, loose cannons.

Six characteristics of SLGs are worthy of note at the outset:
- They are simple and cheap to set up.
- They require significant levels of administrative support.
- They are essentially *clinical* meetings, between specialists and generalists.
- They can produce improvements quickly.
- They bind specialists and GPs together when the market threatens division.
- They have their limitations and these should be recognized.

DIFFICULTIES

This section discusses some of the difficulties that can be expected in developing a system of SLGs.

Obtaining commitment

To be effective SLGs have to be supported by a variety of bodies:
- *Purchasing authorities*: These should see SLGs as a means of encouraging clinicians to agree working practices for themselves. Unfortunately such cooperation on behalf of a District's population may contradict some aspects of a market economy. Hence while fundholding practices increasingly adopt similar approaches to these in discussion with their local consultants, the idea of the collective body of practices doing the same thing for the District's whole population appears to be less well recognized. Yet the principles are the same, and certainly one DHA has supported SLGs since 1990, producing significant benefits to local services at little cost.
- *Specialists*: The increasing understanding of a market economy is proving a useful spur to communication amongst clinicians. Indeed it might be argued that SLGs should not be coordinated within purchasing authorities at all, but within provider units. (There are also powerful arguments against this. See 'Commissioning Working Groups' later.) Catchment GPs would be encouraged to work with their specialist colleagues to find ways of optimizing the services available from that unit. The attractions to a hospital within a competitive environment are obvious and it is perhaps surprising that more Trusts have not developed such collaborative arrangements.
- *GPs*: Obtaining commitment from the broad body of GPs is still harder. Unless they are fundholders they may have little incentive other than altruism to conform to even local agreements, and the first four decades of the NHS have shown altruism to be an unreliable motivating factor. It is also unfortunate that the professional quest for the optimal use of finite

resources should be ensnared within the more contentious debate about clinicians becoming legally accountable for the effect of resource shortfalls. The former can be supported by all factions of the profession while the latter confers grave misgivings upon many. This retards the acceptance of approaches such as that of SLGs.

• *Departments of Public Health:* Clinical effectiveness and cost effectiveness are within the remit of Departments of Public Health, and it should be an early priority of those setting up SLGs to involve their Public Health colleagues. However a difficulty within some hospitals is that these specialists are identified as part of the Purchasing Authority and it may be prudent in the early stages to keep membership of SLGs purely to clinicians from General Practice and secondary care. Later, as confidence in the approach rises, the very real benefits of utilizing Public Health expertise emerge as the threat perceived by some recedes.

If all these bodies feel committed to the SLG approach its inherent simplicity will allow useful change to be brought about with surprisingly little effort. Such commitment will be encouraged by ensuring that tangible, useful benefits addressing GP priorities occur quickly. Achieving these initial 'quick wins' can be an interesting test of health authority commitment to a Primary Care-led NHS.

The dangers of 'medicine by numbers'

To many clinicians the idea of guidelines and protocols is abhorrent. To them it indicates a deep misunderstanding of the complexity and variability of clinical practice and suggests their professional work can be reduced to a set of algorithms of ponderous, step-wise logic. It is not difficult to find ample examples to support such a view. Yet constructed in a pragmatic manner, by local GPs for local GPs, in cooperation with their local specialist colleagues, cognizant of research experience from the literature and elsewhere, guidelines can become a relevant and valuable facet of continuing medical education. They are then a distillate of local, professional wisdom, and when clinicians use that knowledge they not only do their best for individual patients but also make the best use of local resources, so helping others. A logical extension of the concept of locally agreed guidelines is to incorporate them within GPs consulting room computer systems, and this idea is now being developed within Northampton District with one of the major GP system suppliers.

The insistence that it is the GPs themselves who construct the local guidelines is an important safeguard against simplistic analysis of their work. Surveys of patient opinion by many researchers indicate that components of the *art* of general practice consistently come at the top of patients' priorities (for example Cartright and Anderson 1981, Allen 1989). Empathy, time to listen, and kindness are valued aspects of clinical practice, but hard to measure and impossible to put in a guideline! There is a significant danger within medicine of attention becoming focused on the measurable, to the detriment of the intangible. Conversely, defense of the intangible should not be used as justification for failing to utilize objective assessments where these are pertinent and practical, any more than 'clinical freedom' should be used to justify intellectual laxity.

Matters relating to opportunity costs, the setting of priorities, and being a purchaser–provider

If clinicians avoid the issues of opportunity costs and establishing priorities they merely leave such decisions to be made by others. There appears to be value within a national health service in this being a coordinated exercise within the District, rather than one taking place in a piecemeal fashion at practice or individual level. Involvement will cast GPs in a difficult position, particularly as health authorities and FHSAs coalesce into Commissions and the distinction between the purchasing of primary and secondary care becomes less and less clear. If GPs are to play a full part in the commissioning of health services within their Locality or District, they will inevitably find themselves talking on the one hand as a purchaser and on the other as a provider. Here it is helpful to distinguish between *commissioning*, the strategic process of determining the needs and priorities of a population, and *purchasing*, the operational task of translating commissioning plans into time-related purchasing plans which make the best possible use of the resources made available by the NHS, and which inevitably involve rationing.

It is within commissioning that clinicians and colleagues from the health authority have to make choices when setting priorities. Here are the stark realities of opportunity costs, risk sharing, clinical and lay pressure groups, and the evaluation of information from health economists and clinical researchers. A cohesive approach from the District's primary and secondary care clinicians is a valuable goal that will be increasingly difficult to achieve, for on the one hand the market stimulates communication, but on the other it may set up tensions and factions that mitigate against co-operation on behalf of the District's population as a whole.

THREE CASE STUDIES

These examples are taken from the Northampton District experience during 1992.

Overview

Since their inception in 1990 SLGs in Northampton have been coordinated by a representative, District-wide GP Core Group. Individual SLGs were simply established where GPs and specialists together felt there was potential for improving clinical services.

The Core Group meets with the DHA monthly to discuss commissioning and purchasing. In this way there is a direct communication conduit between the SLGs and DHA purchasers through the coordinating GP Core Group. This model has recognized since 1990 that GPs should be at the centre of such communications, leading the local NHS. As a consequence of their pivotal position GPs need to be protected from becoming the envoys of particular departments in secondary care when they meet with the DHA. Partly for this reason the remit of SLGs is to be resource-neutral, making the best use of *available* resources. (The matter of building a case for additional resources for a particular discipline is discussed later under the subject of Commissioning Working Groups.)

ENT

This group consisted of two GPs, two ENT specialists, and a Senior Registrar. It was one of the earliest groups to be formed in the District. The specialists wanted to clarify the cases that could most benefit from their surgical opinion and skills, thereby reducing referrals of low priority and improving access for the remainder. The GPs wanted faster routine access to specialist skill and opinion, particularly for young children with apparent conductive hearing loss and for older patients in need of assessment for a hearing aid. The GPs also wanted clear guidance on who should be referred to ENT, and who should not.

Thus the objectives of the GPs and specialists were mutually supportive, as is usually the case with SLGs. Clearly the District's 150 GPs should make the best possible use of their 2 ENT consultant colleagues. Equally, those specialists should ensure that the service they provide is responsive to the opinions and needs of the GPs. That the former are 'providers' and the latter 'purchasers' is unimportant. It is simply a sensible way of providing health care.

During 1992 the Northampton ENT SLG adopted four objectives:
(i) *To produce and disseminate locally agreed clinical guidelines*
Short management notes and referral guidelines for six conditions were written and agreed within the group. These were then presented and discussed at a lunch-time postgraduate education meeting prior to distribution to every GP in the District.
(ii) *To provide direct access to the hearing aid clinic*
The specialists had the understandable concern that open access might flood the hearing aid department with inappropriate referrals. Referral guidelines were constructed with the assistance of the Audiology Department, and direct GP access introduced. This proved convenient for both GPs and patients, and released ten appointments per week to be used by patients with a greater need for a specialist opinion.

(iii) To rationalize the management of glue ear

One use of the appointments released by the hearing aid initiative was to provide a fast track service for children with apparent conductive deafness who had not responded to a period of conservative management under the care of their GP.

(iv) *To provide direct access to the tonsillectomy waiting lists*

The SLG questioned whether an out-patient assessment was necessary prior to inclusion on the routine tonsillectomy waiting list. Appropriate criteria were identified on a specific referral form. All of these forms were screened by a specialist, and where any doubt existed the patient was sent an assessment appointment for the out-patient clinic. Otherwise the patient was entered directly on the waiting list without out-patient attendance.

This system has proved a remarkable success. In 1993 and 1994 direct referrals totalled 317 and 290 respectively, with 8.2% and 8.3% being re-routed to out-patients by the vetting specialist. Thus over its first two years this simple idea alone saved over 550 first appointments in a single ENT department. Such results suggest that within Northampton at least, routine out-patient assessment prior to tonsillectomy is no longer necessary for patients other than young children.

During 1995 this group is auditing the effect of its guidelines upon GP practice, patient opinion of the service, the effect of direct referrals for tonsillectomy and hearing aids, use of the ENT Emergency Room, and the management of Glue Ear. The results will inform the future work of the group.

Plastic surgery

This SLG was formed by the GP Core Group to consider two opposing opinions:

- That the District had inadequate Plastic Surgery services.
- That existing levels of Plastic Surgery should be reduced as the specialty was seen by some DHA purchasers as one of aesthetic procedures and little else.

In the eyes of clinicians the perceived threat was a further weakening of the District's specialist skills in such areas as hand surgery, the removal of lesions from the face, and post-operative reconstruction.

The group consisted of two GPs and a Plastic Surgeon, and achieved its objective of improving the Plastic Surgery service within the District. Furthermore this change was brought about within the annual contracting cycle, not waiting for the next year's negotiations, and demonstrating how the creation of beneficial change is not necessarily dependent upon the market. The process was conducted in three stages:

- *Developing a shared idea of beneficial change*: The group drew up a list of 9 conditions that present in general practice and which it felt might best be managed by Plastic surgery rather than by other specialties.
- *Testing the hypothesis*: A structured questionnaire was sent to every GP in the District, asking them to state to which hospital and specialty they normally

referred each of the nine conditions. They were then asked the same question assuming equal accessibility and a completely free choice of hospital and specialty.

The results demonstrated that:

- GPs would refer to the same hospitals as they were currently using
- but would shift some referrals towards Plastic Surgery and away from Orthopaedics, Dermatology, and General Surgery.
- *Bringing about change*: In the light of these results a case was made to the District Health Authority for an increase in provision of Plastic Surgery on the grounds of improved quality of clinical care.

Clinical guidelines At the same time clinical guidelines were drawn up to classify the conditions referred to Plastic Surgery into three priorities:

- Urgent
- Standard
- Not normally provided within the District

Care was taken to ensure that the classification applied throughout all clinical specialties by discussion with the departments of Dermatology, ENT, and General Surgery, as well as with GPs at a postgraduate lunch time meeting. (For example if a District does not routinely purchase the removal of tattoos within its Plastic Surgery contract then it is important that the procedure is not available within Dermatology or General Surgery, or via an extra-contractual referral.) The guidelines were then circulated to all GPs in the District in the same manner as those for ENT described above. It was felt important to share with the public the suggestion for overt rationing of the third priority, and the conditions that would 'not normally be provided within this District' were published in the local newspaper. No responses were received.

Conclusion: plastic surgery: The work of this group demonstrated how careful work by GPs can directly influence DHA purchasing. The outcome was a 30% increase in day case Plastic Surgery, brought about within the contract year, and to the benefit of all practices, and all patients within the District. At the time of writing the DHA has not tried to recover the costs of the increase in Plastic Surgery by reducing the volume of the other relevant contracts, though this remains a theoretical possibility. Meanwhile the SLG is auditing the effect of its initiatives, to assess whether the guidelines are influencing GP behaviour on the one hand, and whether the priority categories are influencing hospital behaviour on the other.

Obstetrics and gynaecology

Threatened miscarriage Here the hypothesis was in three parts: that if GPs were afforded direct access to urgent ultrasound investigation their care in the community of patients bleeding in the first trimester of pregnancy would be enhanced; that some hospital admissions would be avoided; and that the savings would pay for the improved service.

A business plan was produced jointly with the hospital and agreed by the DHA. Clinical guidelines were developed to ensure that the patient was correctly counselled and followed-up. Methods of assessing the initiative were established.

The idea was proposed, priced, agreed, and implemented within a total of three months. It is seen by clinicians and patients alike as a success. A subsequent audit reviewed the records of the first 171 patients who had used the facility. The audit also obtained the opinion of the GP involved in each case. The results indicated that:

- 21% of the patients were admitted by the GP following the scan, but that 68% would have been admitted had the investigation not been available.
- In 93% of cases the GP felt that the investigation result had influenced his or her clinical management.
- Within the first year of the service 89% of the District's practices had made use of the service (62% of GPs).

The audit results suggest that 61 hospital admissions were avoided within a period of six months by the introduction of this facility, representing a 'saving' considerably in excess of the cost of the service. Thus all three facets of the initial hypothesis were supported.

A difficulty illustrated by this case is that the savings made by one SLG may surface within the work of another department. This is less than motivating for the specialists concerned! Here, for example, it was the work of the Radiology department in providing the additional ultrasound facilities that produced a saving in Gynaecology admissions. Such anomalies need to be addressed.

Overall conclusion It is an irony of the work of SLGs that by improving services they may increase demand. They can then be seen as self-defeating if their intention is purely to improve access to services (a possible GP's perspective), to reduce workload (a possible specialist's perspective), or to reduce costs (a possible purchaser's perspective).

However if their goal is to provide the best services possible, for as many patients as possible, according to clinical need, then their work can be justified as a major contribution to developing the local health service.

ESTABLISHING EFFECTIVE SLGS:
A STEP-BY-STEP GUIDE

For the sake of brevity the notes that follow are didactic, but that does not mean that they are the only way to establish SLGs, or even the best way. They are merely one way that has worked.

Setting up and planning

As with any innovation the first step is to find a flag bearer, or product champion. This should preferably be a member of a representative body of local GPs involved in the commissioning process. That individual should take the lead and responsibility for ensuring that the SLG concept is successfully implemented, keeping the GP body informed of progress.

Experience suggests that a gentle introduction, the details of which are agreed in advance with all the main parties, is most likely to be successful. Clear paths of communication are required between SLGs, the person responsible for coordinating the initiative, the representative group of GPs, and the health authority. Equally, specialist members will naturally wish to keep their unit managers informed about the work of the groups they are in. Similarly links should be established with the local department of clinical and the Medical Audit Advisory Group (MAAG) in order to facilitate the use of objective assessments to underpin the work of the SLGs.

Resource requirements

Once there are more than a few SLGs there is a need for significant levels of administrative support, including office space, secretarial time, and overheads such as printing, telephone, and computing facilities. Clinical guidelines require preparation, production, and distribution; meetings need to be organized and agendas distributed; and progress of the different groups needs to be monitored and recorded. With increasing interest in evidence-based care, it is important that members have access to the latest information where it exists. It may be convenient to base the SLG administration within an existing department of clinical audit. In Northampton, for example, an additional secretary was recruited for that department to undertake SLG work, and there are now additional audit staff as well.

The funding for SLGs may prove problematical. One solution is for the costs to be split between the purchasers and the provider unit involved in the scheme.

The work of an SLG

The function and duration of any one SLG is decided entirely pragmatically. The form of their work may be loosely described as shown in Table 11.1.

That the exercise is underpinned by audit is not to conform to fashion but simply to use objective assessment for its proper use, the measurement of progress towards goals that have already been agreed.

Once the group has done its work, the results need to be circulated as widely as possible to local practices. Ways need to be found of increasing the likelihood of them being reflected in practice protocols, such as discussion at educational meetings, especially those which are practice based.

Table 11.1

1. GPs and specialists describe their perception of current problems in the relevant service
2. Deciding the work to be done: objectives for the group and methods of achieving these
3. Establishing any objective measures required (e.g. 'before and after' audits to assess change)
4. Undertaking initial assessments where indicated.
5. Undertaking the work; constructing guidelines, altering hospital services etc.
6. Assessing the effect.
7. Agreement of when to reconvene the group to reassess the situation. (Perhaps in a year.)

As with other ideas, SLGs have rightly to justify their existence. Audit is the correct mechanism for such assessment, and the work of SLGs is an ideal priority for audit. Every opportunity should be taken to publicize beneficial change once it has occurred. This is good for morale, good for recruitment, and good for justifying requests for resources.

EVOLUTION: THE DEVELOPMENT OF GP COMMISSIONING WORKING GROUPS

SLGs are a valuable mechanism for introducing communication between specialists and GPs and it has been shown that they can quickly bring about tangible benefits in services. However they are an inadequate means of providing high quality advice to inform purchasing plans. They only involve clinicians and are focused upon particular hospitals and Community Units. This reduces the benefits of the market, and even where they link to the health authority through a representative GP Core Group they inevitably still offer partial advice to purchasers.

For this reason Northampton GP Core Group has further developed the concept into Commissioning Working Groups. These have evolved from SLGs but do not replace them. The Working Groups are used to address the priority areas identified by regular surveys of GP opinion within the District, though the model is equally suitable for use in addressing the priorities of any other agency.

There are three processes that take place in a coordinated manner from year to year, allowing a logical and progressive improvement in the quality of services that is appropriate for the resources available and sensitive to competing demands within the District.

- Developing a shared vision of the optimal service for a given subject. This should be at an appropriate level of high quality while resisting the temptation to specify the unattainable. It may be reviewed annually, but is strategic and largely unrelated to time.
- Gathering relevant information concerning what is already happening, and the resource implications of achieving the shared vision.
- The tactical exercise of obtaining within any given year the best fit of current purchasing opportunities and resources with the constantly changing view of the perceived optimal service.

While SLGs are in essence a means of bringing clinicians together to make the best use of available resources, the Working Groups are more formal tools of commissioning.

Essential building blocks for Commissioning Working Groups are shown in Table 11.2.

Table 11.2

Task

1. Agreement of a priority by local GPs.
2. Formation of a group consisting of all relevant skills and interests, including specialists from major providers to offer clinical expertise where appropriate.
3. The construction and maintenance of a shared vision of an optimal service for the given population, including objective justification of proposals where appropriate.
4. The collation of the required information to establish the current position.
5. The identification of the resource implications of providing the optimal service.
6. The construction of a *timeless* implementation plan to move from the current position to the optimal service. (Speed of implementation is a purchasing decision, not commissioning.)
7. The production of an appropriate report for the commissioning authority in the Autumn to inform purchasing decisions concerning the next financial year.

CONCLUSION

This chapter has tried to demonstrate that specialists and GPs working together within SLGs is not only a part of developing good clinical practice but has a greater chance than before of influencing the local health service. The NHS reforms will only lead to major benefits if clinicians and managers work together, accepting that there will never be sufficient resources to meet unfettered demand completely.

Specialist Liaison Groups are a simple idea. To make the best use of resources, to question, to learn, and to adjust are all elements of any successful organization (Bodel 1995). They have nothing to do with accepting responsibility for a budget; the idea applies equally well to fundholders and non-fundholders. Indeed they allow GPs to influence planning decisions *without* accepting a budget; to do so at the smallest administrative cost consistent with effective working; and to do so within a group that contains a breadth of expertise that could not realistically be reproduced were the GPs to do it alone. SLGs and their offspring, Commissioning Working Groups, facilitate the contribution of clinicians to the commissioning process, a process that will inevitably take place but which will be better for clinical involvement.

At the same time health authorities must appreciate that if clinicians are to work with them they will expect to do so as peers. While authorities hold the ultimate responsibility for their own decisions, GPs will be right to expect cogent reasons for conclusions made, particularly where these differ from the views expressed by the doctors themselves. It may be more difficult for statutory authorities to make this behavioural change than it is for clinicians to adapt to the concepts of resource management within a cash limited service; but it is one they shall have to make.

The chapter has tried to bring together elements of commissioning, rationing, cooperation, the market, resource management, administrative economy, and clinical audit to describe a simple means of helping improve care within the NHS. It assumes the goal to be the retention and development of an integrated, population–based service that aspires to the equitable use of resources to provide high quality, cost-effective services. If that is the case then the ball is firmly in the court of the commissioning authorities to create effective working relations with the clinicians in their area. SLGs and the associated organizational structures described in this chapter, are practical means of nurturing and harvesting that vital crop of clinical opinion.

ACKNOWLEDGEMENTS

My thanks to Janet Poole, SLG Manager, Northampton District, for her help with this chapter, and to Michael Sobanja, Chief Executive of Northampton Health Authority, for his continual encouragement over four years of SLG development.

BIBLIOGRAPHY AND FURTHER READING

Allen, D. (1989). Lay proposals for the development of general practice; a view for the Royal College of General Practitioners Patient Liaison Group. RCGP, London.

Bodel, R. (1995). Everyone a rainmaker. Perceptions of 'The Learning Organisation'. *Insight*. **Vol. 8** Issue 1; Jan–Mar 1995, pp. 21–7. The Operational Research Society.

Cartwright, A. and Anderson, R. (1981). *General practice revisited*. Tavistock Publications, London.

Dunning, M., McQuay, H., and Milne, R. (1994). 'Getting a Grip'. *The Health Service Journal*, 28th April 1994, pp. 24–5.

'GPs Developing Local Health Services: The Northampton Experience'. April 1994. Northamptonshire Health Authority. (1994).

Grimshaw, J. and Russell, I. (1994) Achieving health gain through clinical guidelines. 1: Developing scientifically valid guidelines. *Quality in Health Care 1994*, **3**, 45–52.

Willis, A. (1993). General Practice — A Force for Change. In *The New Face of the NHS*. pp. 179–96 (Peter Spurgeon, ed.). Longman.

Part III

Part III

12 Professional development in the new NHS

Jacky Hayden

In part I of this book the Editors argued for a new approach to continuing medical education which would embrace a much broader concept of professional development. In part II various examples of professional development exercises have been described. In the final section we look at the new NHS and where the future might take us.

Major changes in the way the NHS is managed have taken place since 1990: many of which will influence how general practitioners and primary care teams develop and this is the subject of the first part of this chapter. The second part emphasizes the importance of pursuing the themes that have been promulgated earlier in the book.

DEVELOPMENT IN THE NHS

The health service reforms began in 1990. They were introduced at the same time as a new contract for general practitioners and the unrest among many general practitioners created by this contract masked many of the changes in the early stages. The biggest change was the creation of a purchaser provider split. This split, between those who held the budget and those who delivered health care in the NHS, was a totally new concept. For the first time in the history of the NHS funding of patient care became transparent and, thus, a real issue. With it came the development of acute trusts, which were responsible for providing secondary care, and community trusts which were responsible for providing care in the community. The providers of secondary care, the trusts, were split from the purchasers, the district health authorities.

At the same time, general practitioners were offered an opportunity to hold the budget for patient care. Initially, this was limited to a small number of larger practices which were allowed to manage the budget for a limited range of secondary care procedures. Although no formal evaluation has been carried out there was enough enthusiasm for it to be later extended to include smaller practices, including groups of single handed practitioners. A few leading edge practices have been encouraged to hold the total budget for patient care. In some areas practices have joined together to form larger purchasing consortia, which, because of the size of their budgets, have been able to influence health care providers quite significantly. However, although there has been considerable media coverage of fund-holding, both negative and positive, the district health authorities remain responsible for the majority of the budget for health care.

Prior to the NHS reforms, Regional Health Authorities (RHA) had been responsible for managing the budget for patient services in the region. As more district general hospitals were given trust status the responsibilities of the RHA diminished. In a major review of the management of the NHS it was proposed that RHAs should be abolished, new health authorities would be established and a smaller number of Regional Offices of the central NHS executive would be introduced to develop an overall monitoring role. It was recommended that the new health authorities, sometimes called commissioning authorities, should subsume the roles previously undertaken by the Family Health Services Authorities (FHSA) and the District Health Authorities (DHA). The area covered by some of these new health authorities would have been too small to use finances effectively, so it was also proposed that there should be some mergers across districts, bringing together two or more FHSAs and DHAs.

Regional education and development groups

The RHA had previously taken an important role in funding and monitoring education and training for medical and non-medical staff in the health service: these roles had to be taken over by someone else. The new regional office largely cover an area the size of two RHAs. Each regional office has established a regional education and development group, which is responsible for advising on education and training. If there were a natural home for a regional consultancy in professional development it would be here.

The focus for postgraduate medical education remains with the postgraduate dean's organization (based on the old NHS regions) although the dean and regional adviser in general practice are now partly responsible to the regional office.

In England, the budget for general practice training is held by the Post-graduate Dean and managed by the Regional Adviser in General Practice. In Scotland, there is a Scottish Postgraduate Medical Education Committee, which acts in a similar way to a health authority, and is responsible for purchasing education and training.

Development of educational consortia

Rather than allow each health authority to take responsibility for a smaller budget for training for nurses and professions allied to medicine, educational consortia have been established to take over this responsibility. The education and training consortia bring together both providers and consumers of education and training and include general practitioners as one of the major employers of nurses trained in the health service. The educational consortia will be responsible for setting and monitoring standards for non-medical education, but they will also have an important responsibility for innovation in both medical and non-medical education, much of which could include development of the primary health care team.

It is therefore highly likely that these consortia will have an important effect on professional development in general practice because the future of primary care is dependent on effective teamwork. They should form a bridge where doctors, nurses, and others can explore new ways of working.

Changes in training for specialist medicine

Training for specialist medicine has been revolutionized. The Calman (1993) proposals will result in a shorter, more organized training for specialists culminating in the award of a certificate of completion of specialist training. Many of the underlying principles in the changes to specialist medical training are based on the lead taken by general practice training. Although it is always difficult to predict what effect this might have, it is likely that the doctors will complete this training at a younger age than their predecessors, and may not have the breadth of experience that develops with maturity of a clinician. This focuses attention on the need for professional development to continue after the training has been completed.

Junior doctors have traditionally worked long hours, often with very little rest. At the same time as the NHS reforms were taking place, the number of hours worked each week by junior doctors has been reduced. This has in turn changed the way of learning. Doctors have traditionally learned through an apprentice model, a system in which role-modelling has played an important part. As many junior doctors no longer work for one or possibly two consultants as part of a 'firm', this style of learning has been replaced by more formal teaching.

Education for consultants has changed too. Medical royal colleges have set out programmes of continuing medical education. Some are expecting participation in these programmes in order to retain registration as a specialist.

The changes in the hospital service and in particular the moves to a consultant-run service have meant that many more doctors are currently needed. General practice, like hospitals, is finding it increasingly difficult to recruit and replace colleagues and is having to think imaginatively about alternative strategies.

A PRIMARY CARE LED NHS

The NHS reforms have emphasized the important co-ordinating role of primary care in the care of patients. Professional development of the primary health care team will become yet more important as this co-ordinating role grows. However, a primary care led NHS is not just about primary care and it is certainly not just about general practice. The phrase conceals important changes that will need to occur on the interfaces between primary and secondary care and between primary care and social care. Important changes will also need to occur in the relationship between general practitioners and health care managers.

The purchaser provider split is as much an opportunity as a threat. Too much power and too little sensitivity on the part of general practitioners, particularly those with large budgets, could severely threaten an acute or community trust; unwillingness to use the new found influence on the part of general practitioners could negate the important concepts behind the split. The answer seems to lie in commissioning a carefully planned and co-ordinated approach to developing health care services to meet the identified needs of the population. This approach should allow planned use of the budget and will involve much greater co-operation and understanding across the important interfaces.

The development of evidence based care

Evidence based care is not a new concept. To suggest that clinicians had been basing their care on whim and anecdote is hardly a commendation of our predecessors and teachers. Nevertheless, the NHS reforms have created a climate in which evidence of effectiveness is increasingly important in deciding whether a patient should have one particular course of treatment or another. It is possible that technological developments will give us instant access to information in relation to the effectiveness of different treatments. Before that technology becomes available it will be essential for primary, secondary, and social care to work together to agree the best course of action for a series of different clinical situations. Where evidence is available it should provide an important tool for the development of guidelines.

Currently, much of this evidence is based on experience in secondary care. This may be because there have been more opportunities in secondary care or perhaps because general practitioners have not valued critical appraisal and research skills as highly as some of the other skills that are used in work with patients. This may not be true for other members of primary health care teams and it certainly would not be true of colleagues working in public health medicine.

THE ROLE OF THE NEW HEALTH AUTHORITIES

The NHS reforms have created new health authorities which will be responsible for assessing the health needs of their population, and ensuring, through a contracting and commissioning process, that there is adequate provision of health and social care to meet the identified need.

Quality

Since 1990 the Medical Audit Advisory Groups (MAAGs) have taken an increasingly important role in continuing professional development. In Chapter 2 the importance of audit as a tracking system for strategic plans is emphasized. During the years since their inception, the role of the MAAGs has changed; although they were developed to encourage general practitioners to audit their work they have gradually taken over a role that includes professional development and quality improvement.

As the new health authorities become independent, they will be more autonomous in the way that they develop the role of MAAGs or their replacements. Some may choose to enhance the quality improvement role, while others may promote the role MAAGs to take on professional development. The two roles are obviously not mutually exclusive. Improved professional development is likely to result in improved quality of care. In some areas MAAGs have recognized the importance of a multiprofessional approach to learning and have taken the lead in setting up a primary care education team.

Commissioning of primary care

The purchaser provider split has largely focused on the interface between primary and secondary care. As the new health authorities develop, their managers will inevitably consider how they will commission primary care. They will need to consider what services the population is likely to need and what standards are reasonable to expect.

There has been resistance to any change in the individual contract between health authority and general practitioner, yet few practices offer personal lists, and even fewer operate a system of care which does not involve other health professionals. Consideration is already being given to a contract between health authority and practice, and leaders within general practice are discussing how a practice's performance might be measured. What is certain is that the traditional contract with an individual doctor is likely to be complemented or replaced by alternatives.

One of the strengths of general medical practice has been flexibility. It has been possible to respond to varied clinical and managerial demands with speed and efficiency. Yet, paradoxically, one of the major challenges facing primary care continues to be the inability to ensure consistently high standards of care across varied patient groups. For example, general practice in the inner cities includes some of our best and some of our worst examples of care.

As health authorities take a greater responsibility for assessing the health needs of their population and, ensuring that there is adequate provision, they will need to address areas in which primary health care is not meeting expectations. Some authorities are already beginning to set up alternative models of primary care, using primary care centres, others are augmenting existing services with additional salaried general practitioners. Trusts have recognized the importance of primary care and some are preparing the ground to become providers of primary care as well as secondary care.

Many graduates of vocational training are not ready to enter partnership (Baker *et al* 1995) and working in a salaried system, often with inducements of protected time for education or research, may be an attractive option.

THE IMPORTANCE OF PROFESSIONAL DEVELOPMENT

The changes within the health service will encourage the expansion of primary care, and these changes are likely to be more effective if there is a system of professional development established in primary care, responding to and anticipating change. However, effective professional development will depend on individuals within the health care team and leaders who are able to identify opportunities and encourage good practice. As the role of primary care develops there will be new skills to be learned. In 1986, when the concept of a good practice allowance was being considered, no-one would have thought that general practitioners would be expected to develop skills in managing their total practice budget, or that they would be considering the cost benefits of practice based treatment.

The additional skills required for primary care in the new NHS will need to be learned, often in ways other than the traditional lecture. Although it will be essential for general practitioners to learn alongside consultant colleagues there will be other groups of health professionals who will take an increasingly important part in their professional development. Nurses, health service managers, and colleagues working in social services all have skills which are essential to the expanding role of primary care. Health authorities are likely to adopt an important role in monitoring the education provided by community trusts for members of the health care team. It is important that the health authorities recognize the importance of practice based learning and professional development of community nurses and health visitors alongside general practitioners, practice nurses, and practice managers.

At present, general practitioners achieve their postgraduate education allowance by attending courses and other activities that have received prior approval. Nurses and other professionals have other arrangements. Piecemeal approval for courses will need to be replaced by an approval system which recognizes individual and team development plans and focuses on the delivery of care rather than simply learning activities in isolation.

Action learning

Action learning groups are familiar to many people, even if they are not accustomed to the term. The concept of a group of individuals working together to learn a new task or new skills, is one that has been present in the medical curriculum since the days of the dissecting table, and is continued through the day release programme in vocational training. The idea can be extended to a multi-disciplinary group who are learning new skills fundamental to their role in the primary health care team.

An action learning set usually works with a facilitator. The members of the group will have a common task and are likely to share the need to learn new skills to complete their task. By working through the problems encountered by the individuals in the group the sum of knowledge and understanding is far greater than if the individuals were to work at the task in isolation. The group members also learn skills in problem solving and management of change.

Action learning allows managers and clinicians to work together; by discussing mutual problems, they will understand each others role more clearly. The added benefit is likely to be long standing relationships which develop across practices and across professions. These relationships will often form the foundation of mutual trust and respect which will help move primary care forwards.

Practice based learning

The role of the clinical generalist in the changing health service will become more important as more patient care takes place in the community. It has seemed that highly developed, specialist knowledge has been more highly valued in the past than a broad understanding of the patient, their surroundings, and the impact of their illness on their lifestyle. Continuing medical education has therefore valued the specialist lecture. General practitioners have sat in darkened lecture theatres across the country, desperately trying to remember a string of facts that would help them diagnose and manage a patient with a rare but life threatening condition. Unfortunately, when the patient with the rare and life threatening condition finally arrived in the surgery the knowledge had long been committed to the depths of our memories, and GPs resorted to their well thumbed textbooks.

The changes in the health service have highlighted the importance of high quality primary care to many general practitioners. Those practitioners have set time aside to work with the other members of the health care team to reflect on the service which the practice provides. There may be times when an external expert helps the team to gain new knowledge and skills, but many teams have realized that there is a wealth of expertise within the existing team, although members may find it more difficult to be dispassionate or politically neutral.

The practice as a learning organization

Once practices have developed an ethos of learning from each other in relation to patient care they move towards the concept of a learning organization. In such a practice all individuals work to set and monitor their own standards, within an overall strategic framework. The practice values the contribution of all members of the team, and encourages everyone working in the practice to learn from their daily work. It can be difficult to set aside time for reflection and reading: many general practitioners are only able to find time for reading in the evenings and weekends. It can be difficult therefore to find time to meet as a team to discuss clinical or management issues and learn from each other. The General Medical Council (1995) emphasizes the importance of the patient as first priority, yet there are times when the imperative of clinical work prevents effective learning. Perhaps the solution lies in a practice strategic plan which includes a plan for development and personal education plans, with a system of mentors who will remind us when we are not meeting the targets we have set ourselves.

CONCLUSION

This chapter has underlined the major changes that have occurred within the NHS since 1990. These changes will continue to influence general practice significantly in the years ahead. The important features are the:

- possibility of more interdisciplinary development
- shortage of doctors and the need to develop alternative strategies in primary care
- need to develop greater links and understanding between generalists, specialists, and managers
- need to incorporate evidence wherever possible into primary care
- possible change to the GP contract to a more team based one
- need to develop the practice as a learning organization

The implications for primary health care are profound. General practitioners can no longer assume that their position and livelihood is automatically assured. If they can demonstrate quality, imagination, teamwork, and development they will not only survive but grow to occupy a general role in health care. However, without these qualities, other systems of primary health care, possibly inferior to traditional general practice, are likely to appear. The need for professional development has never been greater.

REFERENCES

Department of Health. (1993). *Hospital doctors: training for the future*. The report of the working group on specialist medical training. Health Publications Unit, Heywood.

Baker, M., Williams, J. and Petchey, R. (1995). GPs in principle but not in practice: a study of vocationally trained doctors not currently working as principals. *British Medical Journal*, **310**, 1301–4.

General Medical Council. (1995). *Duties of a doctor*. General Medical Council.

13   A blueprint for the future

David Pendleton, John Hasler, and Jacky Hayden

The central theme of this book is change and development. The world is changing — not just general practice. Since Alvin Tofler in the 1970s first pointed out that the future pace of change could only accelerate to produce a 'future shock', other authors have continued to elaborate the message.

Charles Handy suggested (Handy 1991) that in our current times — the age of unreason as he called it — change is discontinuous. Change is not merely accelerating as Tofler would have it. 'Step' changes are happening as new technological developments make entirely new things possible. As an example, he cites the speed at which people can travel. Since the dawn of time until the nineteenth century, people could travel at no more than around 25 miles per hour. With the invention of the steam engine, then the internal combustion engine, then the jet engine, and finally the rocket engine, a series of step changes occurred in the speed of travel. The rocket engine made it possible to break away from the earth's gravity and enter space. Now human beings can travel at many thousands of miles an hour — and all in less than 100 years. Handy also includes the telling observation that, in a period of discontinuous change, the past is no longer a guide to the future. The old die confused rather than wiser and more certain.

We do not intend here to raise the matter of whether change really means progress. There is a perfectly sound moral argument that human nature does not change greatly and that this is where wisdom is to be gained. It is also customary at this point for someone to cite the French aphorism 'plus ça change, plus c'est la même chose'. Yet, powerful though these points are, they are irrelevant to our argument here.

The world is changing fast, whether we like it or not. As intelligent professionals, it is our obligation to try to understand the changes we face and react with adaptive rather than maladaptive responses. We may then seek to ignore them, to resist them, or to embrace them.

In this endeavour we are not without guides, though each is speculative and cannot anticipate the next step changes forewarned by Handy. John Naisbitt's often cited *Megatrends* (Naisbitt 1982) was dubbed by the Washington Post 'a field guide to the future'. This book details ten new trends that are changing people's lives in the affluent nations. Several of these have relevance for general practice: the move from centralization to decentralization, the move from hierarchies to networks, and the move from institutional help to self help.

Hamish McRae's *The world in 2020* (McRae 1994) shows how other changes can be anticipated on a macro scale. The world is no longer dominated by developments in Europe or in the United States. The economic might of the Asian nations is starting to change the world balance of power.

To understand these developments is to gain insights into the context in which medicine will be practised in the 21st century. It also allows us to enter that period better equipped for the changes we will have to face, and which some of us may be able to influence.

CHANGE IN GENERAL PRACTICE

In the last 50 years we have seen three step changes in practice. There was the establishment of the national health service (NHS) in the 1940s, the general practice charter in the 1960s, and the new contract in the 1990s. Each of these developments caused a significant rethinking to take place. The last of these was still causing shock waves to be felt for years after its introduction. Predictably, some doctors have attempted to ignore the changes, some have resisted them, and others have embraced them with enthusiasm.

Though each development caused major consequences, none of these changes came completely unexpectedly. Perceptive professionals saw each coming and geared their attitudes to the world as it would be after the change had occurred Perceptive professionals are doing so still. So what might we expect to happen in the future and how will it affect professional development? Though nothing is certain, there are clues to be found in the trends affecting us now.

Society and demography

The people who consult doctors are and will be increasingly well informed. Many are avid readers of health sections of magazines and followers of health programmes on radio and television. Many with particular diseases are members of patient organizations that provide high quality information material. Many are aware of current ethical dilemmas in health care or those which new technology may bring. The challenges for doctors are both in the fields of attitudes and communication skills. The model of consultation tasks developed at Oxford in the early eighties was based heavily on the premise that patients should be involved in decisions about their own health care (Pendleton *et al.* 1984). Those involved in teaching consultation skills know that doctors need to develop their communication skills to be able to share decision making effectively.

Patients are also getting older, and the active work force supporting the elderly is reducing. An increasing number of people will need care and support in the community and primary health care teams will need to decide how they can reduce the likelihood of dependency developing.

Patients' expectations of their doctor's availability have also changed. The citizen's charter and the increased availability of many domestic services have created an expectation of longer opening hours of their local general practice. Out of hours calls are no longer reserved for medical emergencies, deputizing services are able to respond to all requests for visits creating heightened expectations of all general practitioners.

At the same time, the spectrum of disease is changing. Fortunately few young mothers have experienced intrapartum or neonatal death, the infectious diseases of childhood are now largely preventable, the likelihood of encountering severe illness and death are greatly reduced. At the same time the media have created a greater awareness of potentially lethal conditions such as meningococcal meningitis. It is likely that the future general practitioner will need to learn how to help his or her patients live with uncertainty in relation to their health and teach them what signs might constitute serious illness.

Technology

New technology will have a major impact on clinical practice in specialist and generalist medicine and on the relationship between the two. In the former, an increasing number of operations are carried out now by non-or minimally invasive techniques resulting in the need for fewer hospital beds and more day care. One estimate is that by the year 2010, 80% of surgical techniques will be carried out in this way, often by doctors other than surgeons. The people who sleep in hospitals will largely be those in intensive care units or who need hotel care because they lack adequate home support.

Diagnostic activities will become more sophisticated and portable. 'Near patient testing' as it has become to be known will result in diagnostic information travelling electronically to hospital specialists rather than the patient travelling in person. Already it is possible to transmit a visual image of a skin rash to a dermatologist hundreds of miles away, or receive expert advice on surgical technique from an expert in a remote hospital.

Information technology will relieve generalists of part of their handicap when faced with a problem with which they are unfamiliar. The *Oxford Textbook of Medicine* and other data are now available on CD-ROM and are starting to appear in practices, whilst modem links are already in use to link practices with central libraries and databases. Algorithms and decision support systems will be in widespread use on consulting room computer screens. The ability to generate an adequate list of differential diagnoses when faced with a medical problem will no longer depend solely on the doctor's memory. Expert systems will begin to change the role of expert people.

The effect of all this will be to shift significantly the current balance of medical care towards the primary sector. Not only will patients simply not be in hospital but general practitioners will have both the ability and the confidence to deal with many more conditions. This shift has already started with an increasing number of practices dealing with nearly all their asthmatics, diabetics, and hypertensives, to say nothing of major activities in prevention.

Teamwork

Many of the new activities in primary care are undertaken not by doctors but by nurses and administrative staff. In some practices, as much as a third of all consultations are currently carried out by nurses. Experiments are under way on nurse prescribing. Other professions are also appearing in primary care settings, including physiotherapists, dieticians, and psychologists.

The present fragmentation of nurses according to employer will not be sustainable for much longer. There is some evidence to suggest that monitoring and education are better done by nurses. The emerging trend is likely to be that doctors will concentrate more on making diagnoses and problem solving whilst others take over aspects of support, treatment, education and supervision.

Changing roles inevitably create tensions at the interface between professionals. Whilst the hospital services learn to cope with the changing roles between specialists, other tensions may arise between primary and secondary care and between the different professions in primary care. A good example is the difficulties between general practitioners and midwives in some places over who should be responsible for obstetric care.

Nigel Stott and colleagues (RCGP 1996) has defined the core primary care team as those who work within the same building and have described the negative effect in communication when the size of the practice team is increased. It seems that effective health care can only be provided by including the members of the wider primary health care team by working as discrect task based units. As primary health nursing expands, new roles will develop, already some nurses are extending their skills and knowledge through an M Sc. in public health medicine.

Accountability, contracts, and finance

One of the chief causes of unrest amongst general practitioners, since the introduction of the 1990 contract, has been the demand that doctors should be more accountable for their actions. This is not simply a matter of cost effectiveness but a recognition that the service is of variable quality and that primary care of dubious standard is no longer acceptable. At one extreme, doctors may be anxious that they may be found wanting whilst at the other, doctors believe that they are working harder than ever whilst the demands on them escalate. The rise in complaints against doctors has not helped. Yet medicine is not the only activity where more accountability is required. What is happening in health care is a reflection of more general trends in society — paternalism is no longer acceptable.

The success of the purchaser–provider split in forcing secondary care to recognise the needs of patients has not been lost on doctors, managers and politicians. As the concept of jobs for life recedes, it is inevitable that primary care, like secondary care, will come to be purchased through fixed term contracts. It will then be possible for health authorities to negotiate what kind and range of care they want to see. Not only will primary care teams need to agree the content of care but they will also need to demonstrate quality. One of the effects of new technology has been to start making data on activity and quality instantly available.

All medical practitioners base their care on their previous experience and learning. Sometimes the foundations for this care are strong, but in many instances there is little evidence to support one management plan over another. Health professionals are all now encouraged to base their care on evidence from the medical literature; sometimes it can be difficult to see a clear preferable strategy, alternatively we find little published evidence on the topic in which we are interested. As meta-analysis develops, the evidence for one plan of action in clinical medicine should become clearer, lack of conformity to proven national standards will become unacceptable.

It seems likely that all practitioners will undergo a form of recertification in the future and that this will be alongside a system of re-accreditation of the practice. Managers of the health authorities may set the agenda for re-accreditation but hopefully that of recertification will remain professionally led. If recertification is to serve as a developmental process it cannot be linked to the exclusion of minimal competence. It will therefore involve a process of setting and achieving goals or standards; this process will need to be linked to methods that aim to identify learning needs, such as audit including significant event analysis.

A constant source of strife between doctors and politicians is money. It is possible to take any number of views as to what might constitute adequate funding for the NHS. Doctors have to recognize that the tension is the price that has to be paid for working in what is generally regarded as a very civilized health care system. On the one hand the money coming in is limited by the Treasury from direct taxation whilst on the other hand, doctors and others face unlimited demand. Only a few months after the NHS was introduced in 1948, Aneurin Bevan, then Minister of Health, announced to the House Commons that the demand for teeth and spectacles had exceeded all expectations (Klein 1983). With rising costs due to the elderly, new advances, drugs, and increased patient expectations, doctors and politicians will be faced with challenges of significant proportions.

Contracts for the provision of health services may become limited in time. The distribution of work between doctors, nurses, and others is dynamic instead of static. Communication technology continues to advance. Certainly, the pattern of medical care is changing rapidly. For these reasons, the concept of a fixed partnership, possibly for life, with indefinite contracts for staff, may no longer be tenable. The idea that only doctors should be partners in practices will be seen to be out-of-date. Some doctors and nurses will either be employed on fixed term contracts or work in some other way for the partnership (Hasler 1994). Some administrative work will be die away from the practice. The key will be flexibility. The practice will not be set up for life — people will come and go. Handy's own vision for an organization is like a clover leaf (Handy 1991). A central core (a small partnership of doctors, nurses, and managers) develops the vision and plans development. A second section (other doctors and nurses) does work for the partnership on a contract basis. A third section (finance officers, secretaries) supports the organization on an intermittent basis.

General practice at centre stage

Government ministerial statements claiming that primary health care is the central pivot of the NHS are true, not because of policy, but because of some of the changes to which we have referred. Primary Health Care is indeed moving centre stage. Why then does general practitioner morale appear to be low in some places? Possibly it is because stress and anger tend to be the response when people feel that their lives are out of their control. The Government's behaviour towards the medical profession in their handling of the 1990 contract has caused such a reaction.

It is right that doctors and others should be more accountable and financially responsible but the method of introduction of enforced change left a great deal to be desired. There is plenty of evidence to show how change can be introduced effectively (Rogers 1983). Politicians appear to have ignored it with respect to this particular reform when they seemed to get it right in other areas such as the introduction of the compulsory wearing of seat belts. In the case of seat-belts, legislation was not introduced until increasingly powerful advertising had already encouraged a majority to wear them. In the case of the new contract for general practitioners, no such preliminary period was allowed in which many doctors would have willingly changed their behaviour. By treating all general practitioners as recalcitrant, the government alienated the majority.

One particular difficulty stands out — the need for the change agent to have credibility with the group he or she seeks to influence. At a time when doctors are being influenced to provide care that is supported by scientific evidence, it is unfortunate that major upheavals are taking place in the NHS with no clear plans for evaluation (Bloor and Maynard 1994). Similarly, professionals are required to carry out clinical procedures for which there is neither supporting evidence nor a clear professional consensus. Furthermore, as the workload rises, general practitioners believe with some justification that no significant extra resources will follow. General medical services income may be prevented from rising significantly and reimbursements for nurses and other staff may be cut.

UNDERSTANDING AND EMBRACING CHANGE
IN GENERAL PRACTICE

Whereas specific changes are hard to predict, the process of change follows certain predictable patterns. One of these is the movement between simplicity and complexity. Thomas Kuhn (1962) in his seminal work on the nature of scientific change described a cycle from a simple theory, or paradigm, through a stage of increasing complication, to a new paradigm that simplifies again. He showed that anomalies to the original theory's predictions were first undetected, then denied, and then stored as problematical until a new theory or paradigm was suggested which explained the original phenomena and the anomalies. As the old theory begins to be broken down by new discoveries, science is said to be 'between paradigms'.

The 'between paradigms' period is interesting in its own right. The scientists know that the old theory no longer holds but they cannot break away from it. They are not stubbornly holding a theory they know to be false, but they currently still see the world and understand it in these terms. It is not until a new paradigm is defined that they are able to change their perceptions.

The same is true in other fields. John Naisbitt (1982) describes us as living currently in the 'time of the parenthesis' in which we have neither left behind the past nor yet embraced the future. We cling to the known past for fear of the unknown future. Warren Bennis, in his essay 'On the leading edge of change' (Bennis 1993) quotes an essay by Bob Waterman and Ibsen's play *Ghosts*. 'We're controlled by ideas and norms that have outlived their usefulness, that are only ghosts but have as much influence on our behaviours as they would if they were alive'.

General practice may be between paradigms. So may professional development for general practitioners. Yet some of the key features are known and have been outlined above. The salient points raised are elaborated here

Changes in care

It is extremely significant for the practice of medicine that patients are now expecting to share the decision making process with doctors. This is arguably more significant for practice than any change in medications has ever been. It is the end of medical paternalism. The doctor does not know best but, between them, the doctor and the patient can come to a mutually acceptable decision. This style of consulting also produces real improvements in the subsequent adherence of the patient to the recommendations. Involvement increases commitment to the decision and subsequent compliance with it.

Information is the key and everyone will have increasing access to it. As information is more readily accessible by all, traditional medical professional boundaries will erode. General practitioners will increasingly spread their functions into the province of specialists who hitherto had a monopoly on detailed knowledge. Nurses will take over some of the general practitioners' role, in areas to which they are better suited. The flow will not end there, however, as patients will increasingly gain access to the same information. In this way the first boundaries to erode will be inter-professional. Ultimately the boundary between patients and health care providers (usually referred to as 'professionals' because of their knowledge and training) will become more blurred.

In the twenty-first century, medical practitioners will not act as the repositories of knowledge but as advisers on health related matters and, in those countries that have embraced the central role of primary care, as gatekeepers to expensive and/or potentially dangerous procedures. Patients will still consult a healer when in need, as they have down the ages, investing him or her with the power to heal. Yet healers' decisions will be under scrutiny from the medical establishment and from better informed patients who will expect to take part in the decision making process, and to understand and accept reasons given for decisions taken.

Changes in funding and role

No longer is all medical care free to the patient. This dream was always impossible as it could not cope with ever rising expectations of patients and the constant discovery of more esoteric and expensive procedures. Now 'essential' care is free and the definition of essential is elusive. Waiting lists used to be the mechanism for rationing care on the basis of need. Now the purchase–provider split has changed the acceptability of waiting, and made general practitioners themselves ration care on the basis of need. This also changes their role.

Doctors generally consider the needs of patients as individuals. Now they must consider the needs of their practice population as well in order to ensure that funds are well used. Increasingly, explanations may need to be given to patients who are denied access by their own doctors to expensive forms of care. They will need to understand and accept the choices that have to be made in order to make less expensive care available to other people.

If general practitioners are to embrace these changes, they will need to be supported. Doctors will have to adapt to radical changes in their relationships with their patients and their colleagues.

There are additional changes possible for those general practitioners who are willing and able to redefine their role and re-think their involvement with their patients. The local health centre may become more than a renamed surgery. It could easily offer more varied health services, some of which are not far removed from the doctor's current role. There are already health centres offering such services as dentistry, physiotherapy, and counselling. The days when meals on wheels, home help, and slimming clinics are available through the health centre may be closer than many imagine. The really entrepreneurial may introduce a fitness centre, health cookery classes, a healthy-eating restaurant, and a beautician. Naturally these would all be offered on a paying basis.

Bevan need not be turning in his grave at these thoughts, so long as the threat of ill-health is lifted from all equally, but they cannot be ruled out as the basis of funding shifts. They will be resisted by some health professionals too who will find them trivial or exploitative. Yet a health centre may generate sufficient funds thereby to use in many and varied ways — either to enhance the partners' income or to provide additional funds to invest in patient care.

Core, expected, augmented, and potential services

The changes affecting general practice are similar to the changes affecting many organizations that provide a service. They go through a 'cycle' that has been described in terms of the core, expected, augmented, and potential services offered in a competitive market.

The core service is that which defines the organization. For an airline, this is a flight from A to B. Yet soon the discerning passenger comes to expect more than the minimum — inflight meals and entertainment. Airlines competing in these areas alone have to compete on price as all of their competitors offer these services. Augmenting the service with such innovations as personal televisions, phones, and faxes in the air, or a slumber service on evening departures, allows a premium price to be charged. The potential services offered are limited only by the airline's imagination and their funds for investment.

This is also a cycle, as what is expected soon becomes core, and what was introduced as an augmented service soon becomes expected. Similarly, when the entire product has become complex and expensive, providing the original core service at basic cost once again seems attractive.

In the case of the provision of health services, the cycle has barely begun and it is to be welcomed, not feared. The essence of the successful service organization is a satisfied customer who returns to the same organization because of the history of trust that has been established. Such sensitivity to the needs of patients is entirely consistent with good care, though there are inevitable questions to be resolved about the nature of a healthy relationship between patients and health care providers.

THE CHANGING NATURE OF MEDICAL EDUCATION

As medical care changes our attitudes, skills, and knowledge will need to change too if we are not to become out of date and potentially unfit to practise. As we emphasized in Chapter 1, medical knowledge changes rapidly. It may be totally inappropriate for all general practitioners to aim to keep up-to-date on all aspects of medical literature, probably entailing reading more than 200 articles and 70 editorials a month, many of which are based in secondary care.

General practice has now evolved a literature of its own, and has developed skills and values that relate particularly to general practice. Although there may still be a need for expert input into our learning from secondary care, this will become more selective, answering specific issues relevant for general practice. Much more importantly, rather than the random approach of provision of medical education, each practice will begin to undertake a series of activities to identify which areas they need to focus on in their educational programme.

We have already seen the effect of the Department of Health influencing the provision of care and medical education through the Health of the Nation programme. Within that programme and others like it, health authorities will begin to set their own agenda, and use it as a base for their purchasing plans. Practices will relate to smaller populations; purchasing plans may be modified to meet the specific needs of the practice or local population. The patients in the practice may influence the practice agenda too; they may be concerned about specific health issues and may influence the provision of health care through local groups or patient participation groups.

Using information from national, district, and local groups, practices will begin to set a strategic plan of health care activity which needs to be delivered. Each practice will then use audit to identify their current level or quality of care and from the results should be able to define educational need for the practice. Within the practice individuals will decide who will take prime responsibility for each of the new tasks and arrange a series of training events to meet the demands of the new task. All this is achievable in a well motivated practice, but it is much easier with outside facilitation. In earlier chapters we have described ways of facilitating the process.

THE EMERGENCE OF PROFESSIONAL
DEVELOPMENT

As practice changes, so the panoply of related services must also change. We argued in Chapter 2 that audit and continuing medical education were part of a professional development cycle. We also argued that professional development starts with the needs of practices and practitioners (see Chapters 8 and 10). It is logical that the development cycle should start there as these are the people who are closest to the patients — they are the front-line service providers.

The twenty-first century will require that professional development replaces an old emphasis on education. Help is needed across a wide range of needs. The first is help in the formulation of practice strategy, and in the diagnosis of practitioner needs. Help is also required in the development of supplementary practice services, in the introduction of new technology, in the examination of new ethical dilemmas, and the like. This list is merely indicative. The old educational paradigm will be useful in some areas and less so in others.

Similarly, it will make little sense to have an entire machinery for audit separated from the provision of other professional development services. The organizations serving Continuing Medical Education and Audit need to be merged and their role expanded. The concept of a professional development consultancy service (PDCS) has some merit.

Professional development consultancy service

Such a service would be charged with helping entire practices to develop and change, not merely one of their constituent professions. The PDCS would take on many roles. The first would be the provision of help to practices in strategic planning, in which they take a comprehensive look at the services they want to offer and the organization they want to become over the next 5 years or so. This is the establishment of a developmental context in which needs will be identified at the practice and individual levels.

Emerging from these strategic planning exercises, in the ways described by King and Flew in Chapter 3 will be development needs which must be met. Such activities thus guide both the practices and the PDCS. The former knows what it needs, and the latter gains insight into the provision required.

Audit, as described by Martin Lawrence in Chapter 9, would thrive in such a system. It would become a fundamental guide to the effectiveness of clinical care, or of any other change that needs to be monitored as the practice develops.

Other roles for the PDCS may also be anticipated from the other chapters in Part II of this book. It would serve as a resource investigator, networker, and facilitator, bringing together people with needs and those who may be able to help them meet their needs. It would serve as a disseminator of new findings — a communicator and help with implementation. It would serve as a supporter, confidant, and coach.

The PDCS would be staffed by a range of professions — academic and practising doctors and nurses, psychologists, educationalists, researchers. All would share a common goal or mission namely:

To provide consultancy services to health care providers which maximize the impact of primary care on the health of the community

They would all function as consultants who regard the practices in their areas as clients and who seek to serve their needs. (Consultant here is defined as management rather than medical consultant.) They would regard their role as bringing the academic world and the world of practice closer together. They would address the problems of information overload and retrieval, and bridge the gap between new information and behaviour change. They would help to ensure that, where evidence for a course of action was clear, the professionals adopted it. The PDCS would draw on the best that academic research has to offer, helping disseminate it into practice, and also help medical practice set the agenda for some of the research in the universities.

We envisage that there would be one or two such services in each Region. They would comprise a number of basic facilities and staff. An office would be required to co-ordinate activities and provide a convenient point of contact. Its specific location would depend on the other facilities in the Region. Its location and size would be determined not only by the needs to which it was responding but also on these additional and related facilities locally.

The service would be staffed by a central core team and a network of additional resources. The permanent headcount would be small — essentially no more than a senior co-ordinator and a small support staff, though more may be helpful. Its additional resources would come from other local professionals with time to invest. Each would need to have sophisticated technology to help them both deliver the service and stay in touch with the centre. Key consultants would serve the needs of a portfolio of practices with whom they would form long-term client relationships.

Each service would need to set up a network of relevant individuals and organizations. Central to this at first will be the Regional Adviser in General Practice and his or her colleagues. Already, most Regional Advisers see their role beyond the provision of education. Ultimately, the service would come to supersede these more traditional roles or cause them to be reconsidered. General Practitioner Tutors at local level will also need to be an integral part of the service. Many are now experimenting with roles reflecting the activities described in Part II of this book. Collaboration with University Departments of General Practice would be essential. The faculties of the Royal College of General Practitioners should stimulate and facilitate these changes.

It is essential that other disciplines are also involved. In addition to General Practitioners, the Professional Development Consultancy Service would be staffed by a range of professionals — nurses, psychologists, educationalists, researchers. It is also important to recognize the potential contribution of public health as primary care realizes its role in population medicine. All these disciplines would have access to an even greater range of help through their own networks. In this way, they would be able to meet a broad range of needs from technical (architecture, finance, technology) to interpersonal, and clinical.

The PDCS will have a range of learning activities at its disposal. Many of these will be skills-based, some might use advanced computer techniques, others might need the guidance of a local facilitator. All members of the health care team will learn together where it is appropriate. Alternatively, a small multi-disciplinary task force may spend time away from the practice learning with similar teams from others practices, to bring new ideas and skills back to the practice. The current system of accrediting educational events for the post-graduate education allowance (PGEA) may become outmoded. As practice and personal education plans become common place, it is likely that these will be accepted for PGEA on a national basis.

In this way, the PDCS would meet the needs of both purchasers and providers. Its people would need to be skilled in coaching and counselling, in facilitation and in consulting to small organizations. They would become experts in the range of techniques outlined in this volume and elsewhere.

The funding of a PDCS would need to be partial — in order to guarantee a number of key posts — with the expectation that the rest of its funds would come from its ability to market its services to practices who are able and willing to pay for them. In this way, its staff would ensure they offer services that are actually required and valued by its 'customers' the practices. The PGEA — now seen to be an outdated concept based on teachers rather than learners — would end. It could be replaced by a development fund available to all practices. Spending of this fund would become part of the contract between the practice and its paymasters — the local health authority.

CONCLUSION

The future of general practice requires new approaches and new skills, new institutions and new attitudes. There will be some, according to Everett Rogers (1983) who will naturally find themselves drawn to the innovations emerging, and others who are horrified at the thought. Yet the future will require the same values as medical care in the past — the value of health and healing, of expertise and rigour, and of respect and care for individuals. It is a future that is to be embraced with enthusiasm and influenced creatively.

REFERENCES

Bennis, W. (1993). *An invented life: reflections on leadership and change*. Addison-Wesley, Reading Mass.

Bloor, K. and Maynard, A. (1994). An outsider's ,view of the NHS reforms. *British Medical Journal*, **309**, 352–3.

Handy, C. (1991). *The age of unreason*. Business Books, London.

Hasler, J. C. (1994). *The primary health care team*. Royal Society of Medicine Press, London.

Klein, R. (1983). *The politics of the national health service*. Longman, London.

Kuhn, T. (1962). *The structure of scientific revolutions*. University of Chicago Press.

McRae, H. (1994). *The world in 2020: power, culture and prosperity – a vision of the future*. HarperCollins, London.

Naisbitt, J. (1982). *Megatrends*. Warner Books, New York.

Pendleton, D., Schofield, T., Tate, P. and Havelock, P. (1984). *The consultation: an approach to learning and teaching*. Oxford University Press.

Rogers, E. (1983). *Diffusion of innovations*. Free Press, New York.

Royal College of General Practitioners (1996). *The nature of general practice*. Report from General Practice 27. RCGP, London.

Index